Research on Ethics in Nursing Education:

An Integrative Review and Critique

Research on Ethics in Nursing Education:
An Integrative Review and Critique

Mary Cipriano Silva
Jeanne Merkle Sorrell

Series Editors: Linda Moody and
Moira Shannon
Council for the Society
for Research in Nursing Education

National League for Nursing Press • New York

Pub. No. 15-2409

This book was set in Garamond by Publications Development
Company. The editor and designer was Allan Graubard. Automated
Graphic Systems was the printer and binder.

The cover was designed by Lillian Welsh.

Printed in the United States of America

Let us dare to read, think, speak, and write.

John Adams

Contents

Foreword

Research on Ethics in Nursing Education is the third monograph
in a series sponsored and published by the NLN Council for
the Society for Research in Nursing Education (CSRNE). Like
the two previous monographs, it is intended to stimulate dialogue and propose challenges to concerned educators and researchers. The interdependence of nursing education practice
based on research and nursing education research based on
practice is exemplified in this present review.

The study of ethics in all aspects of health care, including
the education of health care professionals, is a major focus of
attention in both the professional and lay literature. While
numerous conferences have addressed the interdisciplinary
efforts of researchers, educators, and practitioners, making
this a popular subject of discussion, a scarcity of research
remains.

Nurse educators have been a vital part of the research ac-
complished to date. Dr. Silva's recent book, *Ethical Decision
Making in Nursing Administration,* is her latest in a productive
career in this field of study. With her co-author, Dr. Sorrell,
and the assistance of doctoral students, Ms. Chop and Ms.
Lewis, Dr. Silva has again added to the nursing literature with
a work of expert scholarship and clarity.

Part I provides the reader with a road map that demonstrates the many choices that were made to produce a concise monograph. This careful description of process provides information that can be foundational for future scholars who are reviewing the state of literature in this field.

Part II provides an integrative review and critique on studies that address ethical considerations in curriculum, students' moral development, decision making, and student and faculty behaviors. These reviews include the general focus of the research, theoretical concepts, purpose, methodology, data analysis, conclusions, and a summary discussion. The cogent analysis of research findings raise pertinent questions about the diversity of methods and the scarcity of theory used in designing studies to date. The summary discussions also provide a synthesis of findings under each of the categories.

Part III is similar in format to Part II and addresses attitudes of nursing students and faculty toward some of the major ethical concerns in health care: abortion, AIDS, aggressiveness of nursing care for terminally ill patients, and patients' rights.

Part IV describes studies related to ethical values of nursing students and faculty: comparison of student values over time, student values and faculty values, students in secular schools versus nonsecular schools, and nursing students and students in other disciplines.

Part V synthesizes the findings of the 39 published studies reported in the monograph and offers recommendations based on the implications of the findings from the studies. The need for common frameworks, terminologies, and research methodologies in this field is described. Empirical research and research programs that build on a series of studies are identified needs. The responsibility of researchers to produce scholarly reports and disseminate their findings through a variety of publications also is identified. Strategies to meet these identified needs are suggested by the authors.

Part VI, the final section of the monograph and a major contribution to those interested in pursuing research, provides a bibliography of dissertation abstracts on research on ethics in nursing education by key concepts, authors, and titles.

We invite readers to use this excellent monograph as a basis for dialogue to address the many questions in the field of ethics that must be explored in nursing education.

Linda Moody, PhD, RN, FAAN
Moira Shannon, EdD, RN

About the Contributors

Mary Cipriano Silva, PhD, RN, FAAN, is Professor and Director of the Center for Nursing Ethics, as well as Doctoral Program Coordinator, School of Nursing, George Mason University, Fairfax, Virginia. She has received several awards for the study of ethics: a National Endowment for the Humanities Award; a Kennedy Fellowship in Medical Ethics for Nursing Faculty; a Visiting Scholar Award at the Hastings Center; and participation in bioethics courses at The Kennedy Institute of Ethics. A recipient of a 1990 Book of the Year Award from the American Journal of Nursing for her book, *Ethical Decision Making in Nursing Administration,* Dr. Silva is currently conducting research on the ethics of scarce resources in nursing administration.

Jeanne Merkle Sorrell, RN, DAEd, is Associate Professor and Coordinator of Advanced Clinical Nursing in the Master's Program, School of Nursing, George Mason University, Fairfax, Virginia. Her research interests include ethical concerns related to physical restraint of hospitalized patients and to comprehension of information for informed consent.

Rose M. Chop, RN, MSN, is a nursing supervisor at Alexandria Hospital, Alexandria, Virginia and a doctoral student/

research assistant within the School of Nursing at George Mason University, Fairfax, Virginia. Her interests in ethical issues are related to moral distress and to the development and education of nurse executives, mid-level managers, and staff members in resolving ethical dilemmas.

Carolyn K. Lewis, RN, MSN, is a lecturer in nursing and a doctoral student/research assistant within the School of Nursing at George Mason University, Fairfax, Virginia. Her interests in ethical issues are related to the availability of community-based services for the rural elderly.

Acknowledgments

The authors thank Frederick Rossini, Vice Provost for Faculty Affairs and Research, George Mason University, for the University Research Grant that made this monograph possible. Likewise, we thank Catherine Randall Benson and Anoush Iskenderian for their patience and efficiency in word-processing major sections of this monograph. We also express our deepest gratitude to Moira Shannon and Linda Moody for the opportunity to share this body of research on ethics in nursing education with students and professional colleagues throughout the country. Last, we thank Sally Barhydt and Allan Graubard from the National League for Nursing Press for their strong support for this monograph.

Part I

Introduction to Research on Ethics in Nursing Education

In this section of the monograph, we state our purposes, as well as the data bases and retrieval strategies we used to identify empirical research on ethics in nursing education. In addition, we define terms, delimit the research, describe validity and reliability measures, and discuss the monograph's limitations.

INTRODUCTION

We formulated two purposes for the monograph: (a) to describe, integrate, critique, and discuss empirical research related to ethics in nursing education and (b) to draw conclusions, implications, and recommendations from the reviewed studies for nursing education practice and nursing education research. Because critiquing of the research was a major purpose, we had a responsibility to discuss both the strengths and weaknesses of the studies described in Parts II, III, and IV. In so doing, we made every effort to be fair—to recognize what contributed to the strengths and limitations of the studies. We also made suggestions as to how the studies might be improved.

Prior to initiating our integrative review, we first provide background information leading up to our research purposes. In 1977, Armiger wrote the first significant review of ethics in nursing. She noted that from 1952 through 1966, only three studies on ethics—all master's theses—were located in *Nursing Research.* Over a decade later, Gortner (1985) wrote a chapter for the *Annual Review of Nursing Research* on "Ethical Inquiry" that included the years 1968 through early 1983. The vast majority of references she cited were expository.

Building on Gortner's work, in 1988, Ketefian (in collaboration with Ormond) authored a monograph on *Moral Reasoning and Ethical Practice in Nursing: An Integrative Review*. The monograph was based on Ketefian's (1989) chapter in the *Annual Review of Nursing Research* on "Moral Reasoning and Ethical Practice." Ketefian noted that there were few published research studies on nursing ethics between 1983 through early 1987; therefore, she had to rely on doctoral dissertations. Of the 31 dissertation abstracts on nursing ethics that she referenced, 13 appeared to focus on ethics in nursing education.

More recently, Chally (1990) published a chapter on "Moral and Ethical Development Research in Nursing Education." Although Chally made a valuable contribution, her work was limited in scope to moral development. Our monograph, therefore, builds on and extends the previous integrative reviews by encompassing all located relevant empirical research on ethics in nursing education.

We begin the monograph with a discussion of data bases, retrieval strategies, definitions, delimitations, validity, reliability, and limitations. We then move on to that part of the monograph in which we discuss, integrate, and critique the retrieved published empirical research on ethics in nursing education. From there we draw conclusions, implications, and recommendations from the retrieved studies. Finally, we present a bibliography of dissertation abstracts on research in nursing education by key concepts, authors, and titles.

To locate research related to the study purposes, we used the following data bases: Bioethicsline, Dissertation Abstracts International, Medline, Cumulative Index to Nursing and Allied Health Literature, and On-Line Computer Library Center. We determined 1970 through 1990 as the search period for the computer data bases because these 20 years represent the emergence and growth of biomedical ethics as a modern discipline. Even though the data bases were searched through December of 1990, some articles that were published in the latter part of the year may not have been indexed until 1991 and, thus, are not included in this review. From out of 36 possible key words, seven were used alone and in combination in the computer searches, as they consistently appeared to be the most valid: education, ethics, morals, values, faculty, students, and nurses. Surprisingly, the key word "research" did not identify any references in any of the data bases and was deleted as a key word. One suggested explanation for this finding is that no one used "research" as a descriptor for the index words in their articles.

Along with the computer searches, hand searches were done on located bibliographies and integrative reviews on ethics in nursing, as well as on the following periodicals (1985 through 1990): *Advances in Nursing Science, Annual Review of Nursing Research, Heart and Lung, IMAGE: Journal of Nursing Scholarship, International Journal of Nursing Studies, Journal of Advanced Nursing, Journal of Applied Nursing Research, Journal of Continuing Education, Journal of Nursing Education, Nurse Educator, Nursing Clinics of North America, Nursing Research, Research in Nursing and Health, Scholarly Inquiry for Nursing Practice: An International Journal,* and *Western Journal of Nursing Research.* Because a substantial increase in research on the topic began to appear in the literature about 1985, this date was used as the starting point for the hand searches. The preceding periodicals were selected because over time they have published research articles on ethics. As periodicals were being accumulated, a bibliographic file was maintained for cross-referencing purposes. The goal was to locate empirical research and state-of-the-art reviews that related to research on ethics in nursing education.

The phrase, *research on ethics in nursing education,* was not always easy to define. Although some studies fell clearly into this category, others were ambiguous. Consequently, we included all located empirical research that focused on nursing students or faculty and on any aspects of ethics related to nursing education. We also included research on ethics in which nursing students or faculty were compared against other groups. Likewise, we included studies in which research on ethics in nursing education was a subpart of a larger study.

With these considerations in mind, we specified the following criteria for the analyzed research: (a) studies must be published and cover the topic of empirical research related to ethics in nursing education and (b) studies must be of sufficient depth and breadth to be critiqued. With the exception of doctoral dissertation abstracts, we excluded unpublished works due to retrieval difficulties and uncertainty about the nature of peer review. Because of the large number of dissertations that focused on educational ethics, we included in Part VI a bibliography of doctoral dissertation abstracts by key concepts, authors, and titles.

We also addressed validity and reliability issues throughout the writing of the monograph. We ensured content validity by obtaining relevant research on the topic through the use of several retrieval methods, including computer searches, hand searches, and cross-referencing techniques. Regarding reliability, we took the following steps: (a) establishing criteria for critique of the research articles; (b) selecting an empirical research article on ethics in nursing education; (c) independently critiquing the article in writing based on the established criteria; (d) comparing our assessments for consistency with the criteria; (e) resolving any inconsistencies through discussion and mutual consent; and (f) following the preceding steps for each part of the monograph to ensure consistency in approach.

The major limitation of the monograph is the possible omission of relevant research on the topic. Ideally, our target population was all research on ethics in nursing education that met the monograph's criteria. However, what is presented here is the accessible population of references that emerged from the computer searches, hand searches, and cross-referencing techniques. Although every effort was made to be thorough, the validity of the monograph is compromised to the degree that relevant studies that met the monograph's criteria are omitted.

A second limitation was the difficulty in categorizing studies into Parts II, III, and IV of the monograph. These categories emerged from the broad, but similar, nature of the studies. On occasion, a study was discussed in two parts of the monograph because the nature of the variables fit more than one part. Decisions regarding both the studies' inclusion in and categorization for the monograph were made by mutual consent of the primary authors.

The description, integration, critique, and summary of empirical research on ethics in nursing education now follows. We begin with Part II, which focuses on the broad category of research on curriculums, curricular strategies, and ethics.

Part II

Research on Curriculums, Curricular Strategies, and Ethics

In this section of the monograph, we review 17 studies related to research on nursing curriculums and ethics, effects of education or ethics instruction on nursing students' moral development, process of ethical decision making, and unethical student and faculty behaviors.

NURSING CURRICULUMS AND ETHICS

We located seven articles that focused totally or in part on research related to nursing curriculums and ethics (Aroskar, 1977; Aroskar & Veatch, 1977; Cassells & Redman, 1989; Cassells, Redman & Jackson, 1986; Killeen, 1986; Munhall, 1980; Winder & Stanitis, 1988). (Since the 1977 Aroskar and Veatch article was derivative, containing the same data as the 1977 Aroskar article but for a different audience, the Aroskar and Veatch article is not discussed here.)

Conceptualization

In late spring of 1976, in cooperation with the Institute for Society, Ethics and Life Sciences (now called The Hastings Center), Aroskar (1977) undertook the earliest published study we located on the nursing curriculum and ethics. No conceptual framework was identified for this study or for any of the other studies cited above, except for the Munhall (1980) article, which was based on Kohlberg's theory. However, in their 1989 article, Cassells and Redman noted that they reviewed ethical models, frameworks, and issues as a framework for their five-year comprehensive national survey on the Baccalaureate Nursing Data Project that was awarded to the American Association of Colleges of Nursing (AACN) by the Division of Nursing, Department of Health and Human Services. Although explicit conceptual frameworks were not included in five of the six reviewed articles, all of the investigators, in varying degrees, included a section on introductions, background information, and/or reviews of the literature.

Purpose

Aroskar's (1977) purposes were (a) to identify how ethical problems and issues were currently being incorporated into baccalaureate nursing programs and (b) to discuss implications resulting from these data. Munhall (1980) was interested in (a) levels of moral reasoning of faculty and of baccalaureate degree nursing students during each year of their program, (b) whether or not significant differences in levels of moral reasoning occurred across the four years of the students' program, and (c) whether or not significant differences occurred in levels of moral reasoning between the faculty and their students. Regarding *c* preceding, Munhall did not make clear whether faculty and students were assessed and compared as two total groups or across academic years. In addition, no research questions were raised about background data on either the student or the faculty groups, yet the majority of reported results focused on these data. Munhall was aware of the limitations the research questions posed for her sample, method, and instruments.

Both the Cassells, Redman, and Jackson (1986) study and the Cassells and Redman (1989) study were outgrowths of the previously noted Baccalaureate Nursing Data Project. Some of the data in this project focused on ethics. In the 1986 article, the following major purposes related to ethics were not noted by the investigators but could be inferred from the results: (a) to describe generic baccalaureate senior nursing students' identification of ethical dilemmas they encountered in their clinical practice, (b) to determine the ethical competencies developed by these students to confront ethical dilemmas in their practice, and (c) to determine sources that contributed to the students' ethical decision-making skills.

In the 1989 article, Cassells and Redman defined their overall goal as identifying those ethical activities and responsibilities that define the role of the nurse as a moral agent. As with the 1986 article, the following major objectives were not noted by the investigators but were inferred from the results: (a) to describe 1987 RN senior baccalaureate nursing students' identification of ethical dilemmas they encountered in their clinical practice; (b) to determine the ethical competencies developed by RN senior baccalaureate nursing students to confront ethical dilemmas in their practice; and (c) to compare, at the beginning versus the end of their programs, 1987 RN senior baccalaureate nursing students' reports on their preparation to take actions or formulate activities when confronted with ethical dilemmas in their clinical practice.

Killeen (1986) took a different approach to ethics and the nursing curriculum than did the preceding investigators. She systematically assessed nursing fundamentals texts to identify the presence or absence of any content on ethics and ethical decision making. Although the study was creative, she could have stated her research purpose more succinctly and clearly. Finally, Winder and Stanitis (1988) surveyed both undergraduate university schools of nursing and graduate schools of public health to determine content in these curriculums related to nuclear war. Although their overall purpose was clear in the abstract, it was not clear in the article itself. In addition, specific research questions were not raised until the data analysis. However, all the reviewed studies did add valuable information to curriculum development and ethics.

Methods

Design. Five of the six studies related to nursing curriculums and ethics were descriptive in nature; the sixth study

(Munhall, 1980) was cross-sectional and involved both descriptive data and inferential statistics. The following investigators used descriptive surveys: Aroskar (1977); Cassells, Redman, and Jackson (1986); Cassells and Redman (1989); and Winder and Stanitis (1988). In contrast, Killeen (1986) used predetermined criteria to describe the presence or absence of ethics and ethical decision making in nursing fundamentals textbooks. In addition, she used a correlational design to describe the relationship between year of publication and average number of pages on ethics content for that year.

Sample. In the Aroskar (1977) study, the sample (or perhaps the population, as this information was not specified) was composed of deans or curriculum coordinators in 209 accredited baccalaureate nursing schools in the United States. From these schools, 86 (41%) respondents returned the questionnaires. Aroskar did not specify how the 209 nursing schools were selected, nor did she give a rationale for why deans *or* curriculum coordinators were chosen to be respondents. A second mailing most likely would have increased her rather low questionnaire return rate. Despite these limitations, Aroskar's study provided nursing with valuable baseline data about ethics in nursing curriculums during the mid-1970s.

Munhall's (1980) sample was composed of the following members of baccalaureate degree nursing students across the four years of the curriculum: (a) freshman ($n = 76$), (b) sophomores ($n = 60$), (c) juniors ($n = 81$), and (d) seniors ($n = 88$). In addition, 15 faculty also comprised the sample. The data-generating sample was comprised of 92% of the students and 80% of the faculty. Munhall was one of the few investigators to describe her sampling techniques, albeit incompletely. She used representational sampling for each academic year to obtain a meaningful and adequate sample size for students, and she used proportional sampling for faculty respondents.

In the 1986 Cassells, Redman, and Jackson study, both a sample of generic baccalaureate nursing programs and of students were selected. The program sample was drawn from the AACN member institutions that had previously responded to requests for information from the AACN's Institutional Data System. Based on these criteria, 270 schools constituted the study universe, and 220 deans from these schools returned the survey (81% return rate). The student sample was drawn from the study universe and consisted of all generic baccalaureate senior nursing students who were enrolled full-time and born in September. The number of students who returned the survey was 749 out of 960 (78% return rate).

Although it appears that the preceding investigators gave careful thought to sample selection, we raised the following questions because they seemed unclear to us in the 1986 article: (a) Were students included from schools where deans did not return the surveys? (b) What was the rationale for the September birthdate? (c) Which surveys did what groups receive? In addition, it would have been helpful if the authors specified the number and percent of all generic baccalaureate nursing programs in the United States and, of these, what number and percent were AACN member institutions who met the study criteria. These data would have allowed the reader to reflect more accurately on the generalizability of the study results.

Because of the nature of Cassells and Redman's 1989 article (both expository and research oriented, and including both an RN senior baccalaureate nursing student group and a generic baccalaureate nursing graduate group), the samples were difficult to follow throughout the article. Since deans were not the focus of this article, sampling related to them was appropriately omitted. Sampling criteria were reported as follows: (a) The students were seniors in participating schools (742 RN students and 1467 generic students); (b) those asked to participate had birthdays in September; and (c) if students did not have this birthmonth, they were chosen by random number tables. No mention of the use of random number tables was noted in the 1986 article. For the 1989 article, the investigators could have strengthened their sampling procedures by specifying the procedures that they used for their 6- and 12-month follow-up of generic graduates.

In Killeen's (1986) study of ethics in nursing fundamentals textbooks, a discrepancy occurred between the abstract and the body of the article. The investigator stated in the abstract that 42 nursing fundamentals texts published from 1965 to 1985 were included in the study; whereas, in the body of the article, she stated that the years were from 1960 to the present. Apart from this discrepancy, all fundamentals texts from three major university libraries during one of the preceding time periods were included in the study. Each library served different types of nursing and/or medical programs. Killeen did not state any rationale for the time frame and the variety of universities selected.

Finally, in looking at nuclear issues in curriculums of nursing and public health programs, Winder and Stanitis (1988) selected as their population (their terminology) the 492 undergraduate schools of nursing across the United States that were accredited, and 23 graduate schools of public health that were members of the Association of Schools of Public Health. Of the 492 nursing schools, 240 responded to the survey (49% return rate) from six regions throughout the country. The largest response came from the west north central region (22%) and the smallest response from the southwest region (4.5%). The names of the states that constituted each of the six regions were not noted. Such data, although cumbersome, would have provided a clearer picture of the geography from which the sample was drawn.

Regarding the public health schools, 20 of the 23 schools queried responded (87% return rate, although the article noted an 88% return rate). No regional breakdown was given so the location of these schools are unknown. The investigators did not discuss why a discrepancy existed between the small number of public health schools selected and the large number of nursing schools selected for participation, nor did they offer any explanation for the high return rate for the public health schools and the much lower return rate for the nursing schools. In addition, no rationale was given for use of undergraduate schools of nursing and graduate schools of public health.

Instruments. Aroskar (1977) noted that questionnaires were used in her study but gave no further information about the questionnaires. Considering that the study was published in a nonresearch journal in the mid-1970s, this approach was not atypical. During the early and mid-1970s, methodological aspects of research were often downplayed in nonresearch journals and results were highlighted.

Munhall (1980) used the following three instruments in her study related to the moral reasoning of students and faculty: (a) the Defining Issues Test (DIT), (b) a faculty data sheet, and (c) a student data sheet. Although Munhall described the DIT in considerable depth, she presented no validity or reliability data about the instrument. In her study, the DIT D score (preference for principled reasoning over conventional or post-conventional reasoning) was used appropriately to measure the research questions that focused on levels of moral reasoning of students and of faculty. The stage score of the DIT was also used but its use was difficult to discern in the article. The faculty data sheet and student data sheet contained the following information: age, grade point average (students only), previous nursing experience, perception of moral ethical considerations in nursing content, role of religion, economic level, parents' occupation, and post-high school educational history.

In the 1986 article, Cassells, Redman, and Jackson reported that a Project Advisory Committee composed of deans of generic baccalaureate nursing programs throughout the United States refined and reviewed the surveys to increase content validity. In addition, other deans, students, and recent graduates also reviewed the surveys to increase clarity. The preceding steps strengthened the validity of the surveys; however, the investigators did not discuss reliability. In the 1989 article, Cassells and Redman referred the reader to one report and two previously published articles that detailed the study method. As a result, instrumentation was not discussed in this article. Because of the type of journal in which the study was published, we feel that this was appropriate, especially since the investigators gave interested readers the references they would need to obtain details about the study surveys.

Winder and Stanitis (1988) also used a questionnaire to obtain their data on nuclear education. They described the purpose of the questionnaire and the number of items it contained. They noted that the questionnaire was adapted from an International Physicians for the Prevention of Nuclear War Survey Form. Nevertheless, the investigators did not discuss the nature of the adaptation, nor did they mention validity or reliability of the instrument.

Unlike the preceding investigators, Killeen (1986) did not use a survey instrument; instead, she established the following three plausible criteria to assess the ethics content of the 42 nursing fundamentals textbooks she located: (a) inclusion of the 1976 American Nurses' Association's (ANA) *Code for Nurses with Interpretive Statements* (hereafter referred to as the *Code for Nurses*) and/or the 1973 International Council of Nurses' (ICN) *Code for Nurses: Ethical Concepts Applied to Nursing,* (b) interpretive statements or discussion of the *Code* with inclusion of examples, and (c) guides for ethical decision making. We were unclear about whether one or both *Codes* were used in *b* preceding. We assumed that the 1976 ANA *Code for Nurses,* rather than the more recent 1985 *Code,* was used because the latter *Code* was published after the data were analyzed. However, both the ANA and the ICN *Codes* were incompletely or incorrectly referenced at the end of the article and the ANA *Code* was incorrectly titled in the text.

Data Analysis, Results, and Conclusions

Aroskar study.   In the Aroskar (1977) study, 86 deans or curriculum coordinators (out of 209 accredited baccalaureate nursing programs in the United States surveyed) responded to the questionnaire on ethics in the nursing curriculum. Descriptive statistics were used, and major results were as follows: (a) None of the programs had a faculty member with the term *ethics* as part of an academic title, although six programs had faculty who spent 50% or more of their time teaching ethics; (b) six programs required a course on ethics, and a majority of respondents reported that ethical aspects were integrated throughout their curriculums; (c) the courses that dealt with ethical issues the most were community health nursing, research, leadership, and issues and trends; (d) the most common method for teaching ethics was use of audiovisual material; (e) a vast majority of respondents favored a multidisciplinary approach and viewed incorporation of ethics into a broader program such as "nursing and humanities"; (f) respondents identified professional codes of ethics as the top priority for curricular study; and (g) a majority of respondents saw a need for further development of ethics education in their programs. Also of interest was a comment that a book on ethics in nursing was needed. Since Aroskar's study was published, several such books have been published.

Cassells, Redman, and Jackson study.   As we will see in the Cassells, Redman, and Jackson (1986) study, other curricular aspects also have changed. Of the generic senior baccalaureate nursing students who participated in the study, nearly 75% responded that they were adequately prepared to make ethical decisions in clinical practice. On one-year follow-up, 72% of the former students who responded to the follow-up questionnaire reported being involved in ethical issues in their clinical practice. Most frequently involved ethical dilemmas were patients refusing treatment, caring for patients with a poor prognosis, and resuscitation or stopping of lifesaving treatment. When confronted with ethical dilemmas in their practices, former students were most prepared to (a) identify the ethical aspects of nursing care, (b) use appropriate staff and resources to clarify and resolve the dilemma, and (c) gather pertinent data related to an ethical issue. On the other hand, former students were least prepared to (a) apply laws governing nursing practice to the issue, (b) consciously apply the *Code for Nurses* to their actions, and (c) use an ethical framework to assess and resolve the dilemma. Both prior to graduation and one year afterward, the respondents ranked nursing courses as contributing most to the development of their ethical decision-making skills, although approximately 25% of the respondents did not agree with this ranking. The investigators concluded that content in ethics is being taught in baccalaureate nursing programs.

Cassells and Redman study.   In the 1989 Cassells and Redman study, the primary focus was on the RN baccalaureate nursing student. For these students, the most frequently involved ethical dilemmas encountered in clinical practice were issues of informed consent, resuscitation or stopping of lifesaving treatment, and caring for patients with a poor prognosis. The data regarding these important ethical dilemmas were difficult to interpret because, in the 1986 article, percentage of respondents (generic student graduates) was reported; whereas, in the 1989 article, mean scores of respondents (RN students) were reported.

This difference in reporting of data (i.e., percents versus means) also occurred with preparedness of RN students to take action when confronted with an ethical dilemma. In addition, in the 1989 article, but not in the 1986 article, preparedness for RN students was reported both for the beginning and the end of the program. Using t tests to assess differences between these two time frames, the investigators found a statistically significant difference ($p < .001$) regarding preparedness to take action when confronted with an ethical dilemma for each of the 12 listed actions. The results of this and the preceding study are valuable in assessing the nature and degree of ethics content in baccalaureate nursing curriculums between 1984 and 1987—the dates in which the reported study in the two articles was carried out.

Munhall study. Data analysis in the Munhall (1980) study included descriptive statistics and analysis of variance. Major results were as follows: (a) The average level of moral reasoning for baccalaureate nursing students was at the conventional level and for nursing faculty was at the principled level; (b) the four academic levels of the curriculum did not significantly affect students' moral reasoning on the D and stage scores of the DIT; (c) nursing students and faculty differed significantly on moral reasoning as measured by the D scores of the DIT (i.e., faculty had higher levels of moral reasoning than did students); and (d) the higher the students' grade point average, the higher their level of moral reasoning. In computing the results, Munhall systematically addressed her four stated research questions, but did not include statistical values or levels of significance; these data would have strengthened the study by differentiating results from conclusions. Nevertheless, in her discussion, Munhall addressed her framework (Kohlberg), albeit briefly, and also implicitly discussed some implications of her results for nursing curriculums.

Winder and Stanitis study. Winder and Stanitis (1988) appropriately used descriptive statistics to assess nuclear education content in nursing and public health curriculums. Nine of the 20 schools of public health that responded to the survey indicated that some activity concerning nuclear war was part of their curriculums. Specifically, nuclear education

in schools of public health included such offerings as (a) nuclear issues as part of certain courses and (b) electives
addressed entirely on the topic of nuclear war and health.
Teaching methods included such activities as student logs/di-
aries, letters to editors, and talks to public groups sponsored
by students.

Eighty-five of the 240 schools of nursing that responded to
the survey indicated that activity concerning nuclear war was
part of their curriculums. Specifically, nuclear education in
schools of nursing included such offerings as (a) nuclear issues as part of a required course and (b) nuclear issues as part
of nursing and non-nursing electives. Teaching methods included such activities as interdisciplinary lecture series and
seminars. Data from both groups were difficult to discern
because they were reported in summary format, with no clear
linkage to the research purposes. In addition, our calcula-
tions of numbers and percents frequently varied from those
reported, making the conclusions tenuous. Nevertheless, we
feel this topic is important in both nursing and public health;
therefore, more research related to nuclear war education in
nursing is needed.

Killeen study.   In Killeen's (1986) study, data analysis
primarily included descriptive narratives and correlations.
Killeen reported the following results on ethics content in
nursing fundamentals books: (a) Of the 42 textbooks assessed, 45% contained no guidelines for ethical decision making, no code of ethics for nurses, and no discussion of the
Code or its interpretive statements; and (b) a significant correlation ($r = 0.59$, $p < .005$) existed between the year of
publication and the average number of pages of ethics content. Killeen appropriately concluded that, overall, there is a
lack of content on ethics in nursing fundamentals textbooks,
but that content about ethics in these texts has increased in
recent years. As with several of the other studies, we found
the data somewhat difficult to interpret because categories
were not always mutually exclusive. However, the table in

which Killeen presented all 42 texts in relation to the assessment criteria was well-organized and helpful in obtaining an overall picture of the results.

Summary and Discussion

Taken together, the six reviewed studies on nursing curriculums and ethics suggest the following:

1. Investigators used few theoretical or conceptional frameworks as a basis for their research.

2. Overall, study purposes varied widely among investigators.

3. Investigators conducted few comprehensive or long-term studies that assessed the overall curriculum and ethics.

4. Sample size and type of sample varied considerably across studies. Sampling techniques were detailed in some studies more than others; however, overall, the sampling techniques used and the rationales for their use were hard to discern.

5. Overall, validity and reliability measures of the study instruments were omitted or not described in depth.

6. Descriptive statistics were the dominant method of data analysis.

7. None of the studies were published in research journals; rather, the emphasis was on journals that focused on education and clinical content.

In reviewing the preceding summary, we find it ironic that the typical nursing research studies on the curriculum and ethics lacked theoretical or conceptual frameworks. This irony is the result of the commitment nurse educators have made to the importance of theoretical or conceptual frameworks as underpinnings for nursing curriculums at both undergraduate and graduate levels. We wonder why this duplicity between curriculums and research occurs and what can be done about it.

The preceding summary also highlights the lack of systematic research in the area of nursing curriculums and ethics. The variations in study purpose, sample size, type of sample, and diversity of instruments made comparisons and general conclusions difficult. Yet, a systematic state of the science on ethics in nursing curriculums from baccalaureate through doctoral study is essential for both short- and long-term curricular planning. In addition, funding agencies and investigators need a stronger commitment to curricular research on ethics to gain further baseline data between and among curricular levels, so that a sound basis for the incorporation of ethics into nursing curriculums can occur.

EFFECTS OF EDUCATION OR ETHICS INSTRUCTION ON NURSING STUDENTS' MORAL DEVELOPMENT

We located five published studies (Felton & Parsons, 1987; Frisch, 1987; Gaul, 1987, 1989; Mustapha & Seybert, 1989) that focused primarily on the effect of education or ethics instruction on nursing students' moral development. (Since Gaul's 1989 article is a shortened derivation of her 1987 article, it is not detailed here.) All four studies detailed herein were published since January, 1987, in the *Journal of Nursing Education;* however, research on this topic has been published earlier in dissertations (see Part VI of this monograph).

Conceptualization

In all four studies, the investigators' review of the literature focused on both study variables and on Kohlberg's theory of moral development. In addition, two of the studies (Felton & Parsons, 1987; Gaul 1987), explicitly stated that Kohlberg's theory served as part of their conceptual framework. In the Felton and Parsons (1987) study, Kohlberg's early work on levels of moral reasoning was identified and defined, but the investigators did not clarify how these levels helped guide the study or explain relevant results. A discussion of the strengths and limitations of Kohlberg's theory would have strengthened their study.

Gaul (1987) conceptualized Kohlberg's theory based both on his early and more recent works. She identified his three levels of moral reasoning and discussed his six stages of moral judgment, including some of Kohlberg's analysis of the limitations of his own work. Like Felton and Parsons, Gaul did not demonstrate how Kohlberg's theory guided her study or helped explain her results. In addition, to frame her study, Gaul (1987) also used the American Nurses' Association's 1976 *Code for Nurses* (which she refers to as the *Code of Ethics* and incorrectly dates as 1977 in her references). A strength of Gaul's study was that she appropriately linked the *Code* to the study instrument and the discussion of results.

Felton and Parsons (1987) also linked Heider's attribution of responsibility construct, which contains five levels of responsibility in decision making, to the Attribution of Responsibility Instrument, the study results, and the conclusions and implications. The investigators did not discuss why they were unable to clarify the use of Kohlberg's theory throughout their study.

Frisch (1987) and Mustapha and Seybert (1989) discussed Kohlberg's theory as a part of their review of the literature. Kohlberg's theory was used to define moral development in the Frisch study and to establish convergent construct validity in the Mustapha and Seybert study. Frisch primarily focused on value analysis (a six-step decision-making process) as her implicit conceptual framework, while also noting the limitations regarding the generalizability of Kohlberg's theory. In sum, all four studies, whether explicitly or implicitly, used research findings and theory as background information. However, the degree to which research findings and theory were integrated throughout the studies varied considerably.

Purpose

Overall, the Felton and Parsons (1987) study focused on the level of nurses' formal education on ethical decision making. The investigators formulated two hypotheses: (a) undergraduate and master's nursing students would differ significantly on attribution of responsibility and on ethical/moral reasoning and (b) the two groups would also differ significantly on number of dilemmas resolved. Felton and Parsons could have strengthened their hypotheses by making the reader aware that course work was controlled at 18 semester hours for both undergraduate and master's nursing students.

In contrast to Felton and Parsons (1987), who focused on level of formal education as their independent variable, Frisch (1987) focused on a specific teaching strategy—value analysis—to teach ethics content to junior-level baccalaureate nursing students. She hypothesized that the value analysis strategy would significantly impact on these students' level of cognitive moral development. Although this hypothesis made the author's intent clear, only one level of the independent variable was noted; that is, the reader was clear on the treatment for the experimental group but not for the control group.

Gaul (1987) took an approach somewhat different from both Felton and Parson (1987) and from Frisch (1987). Rather than focusing on level of formal education or on a specific teaching strategy, she looked at the effect of an ethics course on baccalaureate nursing students' ethical choice and action. Specifically, she raised two clearly stated questions: (a) Will baccalaureate nursing students who have completed a nursing ethics course demonstrate a significant relationship between ethical choice and action in contrast to those baccalaureate nursing students who have not completed the course? (b) Will a difference occur in ethical choice and action in baccalaureate nursing students who have completed a nursing ethics course and those who have not?

Mustapha and Seybert's (1989) research differed from the preceding three studies in that, in addition to an undergraduate nursing student group, two liberal arts undergraduate non-nursing student groups were also studied. The primary purpose of their research was to determine the effect of type of student (nursing or liberal arts) and type of curriculum (traditional or integrated) on students' level of moral reasoning (preconventional or conventional versus principled). Although the study purpose and rationale for the study were included in the article, they were difficult to grasp from the written text.

Methods

Design. In the preceding published articles, none of the investigators identified their study designs. All designs, however, appeared to be ex post facto, pre- or quasi-experimental, because the investigators used preexisting groups, and/or did not pretest (except in Frisch's study), and/or did not use random assignments to groups. In reviewing the studies, we believe that some of the preceding steps were not feasible (especially random assignment) despite the various threats these designs pose to internal validity. However, other than Frisch (1987), none of the investigators explicitly stated the threats to internal validity caused by their design.

Sample. Student nurses constituted the sample in all of the preceding studies except for the Mustapha and Seybert (1989) study in which liberal arts students also were included. In the Felton and Parsons (1987) study, the data-generating sample was composed of 227 female senior baccalaureate nursing students (out of 361 who received questionnaires) and 111 female master's nursing students (out of 184 who received questionnaires). From a population of 11 nursing schools in the southern United States, the preceding students were selected from one of six schools of nursing. Each school of nursing met the following carefully delineated criteria: (a) National League for Nursing (NLN) accredited programs, (b) state-supported, (c) 50 or more female senior nursing students, (d) 20 or more female master's students, and (e) completion of 18 semester hours of course work.

Gaul's (1987) respondents, who were enrolled at one private university, were comprised of 37 baccalaureate nursing students who were in their second semester of their junior year or who were seniors. Of the total, 17 students who were enrolled in a three-credit elective nursing ethics course constituted the experimental group, and 20 students who did not enroll in the course but were matched with the ethics students for placement in the curriculum constituted the control group. The precise nature of the control group as described was not clear; however, Gaul noted both the limitations of the small sample size and the use of one university on the generalizability of the study results.

As with Gaul's (1987) sample, Frisch's (1987) sample also was small—52 junior students enrolled in a mental health nursing course during the fall or spring semesters at a state university. Of the total, 28 students constituted the experimental group, who not only received the standard mental health course in the fall but also the value analysis strategy for teaching ethics; and 24 students constituted the control group, who received only the standard mental health nursing course in the spring. Like Gaul, Frisch also noted the lack of generalizability of the study results due to the small sample size.

Finally, in the Mustapha and Seybert (1989) study, the sample was comprised of 266 undergraduate students who were enrolled in a small liberal arts college in the midwest. The undergraduate students were composed both of nursing and liberal arts students who had enrolled in either a traditional liberal arts curriculum or in an integrated curriculum (Foundations for the Future) with a focus on decision making as central to both values and moral choice. The number of nursing students in the traditional curriculum was 78 while the number of liberal arts students in the traditional curriculum was 120. Liberal arts students in the integrated Foundations for the Future curriculum numbered 68.

Overall, in assessing the sample characteristics across the four studies, we noted the following trends: (a) the populations from which the samples were drawn were not mentioned; (b) the concept of power analysis to determine sample size for desired effects was not mentioned; (c) the rationale for sample size, type of subjects, and nature of included institutions was not noted; and (d) the type of sampling was not noted, with the exception of the Mustapha and Seybert (1989) study in which the investigators stated that they used a convenience sample.

Instruments. In the Felton and Parsons (1987) study, the Defining Issues Test (DIT) and the Attribution of Responsibility Instrument (AR) were used. The DIT, based on Kohlberg's theory of moral development, is an objective test consisting of six hypothetical stories about a moral dilemma in which subjects respond to questions about the actions of characters in the story. The DR score of the DIT appropriately operationalized the dependent variable of degree of ethical/moral dilemma resolution, and the D score of the DIT appropriately operationalized the dependent variable of level of ethical/moral reasoning. Felton and Parsons were careful to report both strengths and weaknesses regarding validity with the DIT in the past. It was unclear whether the Cronbach's alpha of .79 reported on the D score was obtained by Felton and Parsons or by past investigators. A strength related to instrumentation was the investigators' inclusion of scoring data for both the D and DR components of the DIT.

Although not stated clearly in the article, the Attribution of Responsibility Instrument was apparently developed by Felton and Parsons (1987) to measure the constructs of commission, foreseeability, intentionality, and levels of justifications regarding responsibility. Content validity was obtained by two social psychologists and was assured. In the study, the investigators were careful to establish their own reliability. Both Cronbach's alpha (reliability coefficient of .85) and test-retest reliability (reliability coefficient of .63) were obtained.

Frisch (1987), in measuring the dependent variable of level of cognitive moral development, also used the DIT. She noted that Cronbach's alphas were in the high .70s, that test-retest reliabilities were in the high .70s or .80s, and that criterion validity appeared adequate. The DIT scores used in Frisch's study were the P score (which represents level of principled thinking at Kohlberg's stages 5 and 6) and the stage score (which represents at which stage in Kohlberg's theory subjects' responses tend to cluster). Frisch demonstrated consistency between her implicit conceptual framework of Kohlberg's theory of moral development and the DIT. In addition, Frisch noted several limitations of Kohlberg's theory and of the DIT.

As with the previous two studies, Mustapha and Seybert (1989) also used the DIT to measure levels of moral reasoning among undergraduate nursing and undergraduate liberal arts students enrolled in a traditional or an integrated curriculum. As in the Felton and Parsons (1987) study, the D score of the DIT was used; in addition, as in the Frisch (1987) study, the P score of the DIT was used. Adding to the previously noted validity and reliability data, Mustapha and Seybert specifically reported that convergent construct validity between the DIT and Kohlberg's Moral Judgment Interview was satisfactory and that correlations with a variety of other constructs such as personality and aptitude measures were in the .40 to .60 range. Two other instruments were used in this study: the Demographic Data Questionnaire and the Shipley Institute of Living Scale, which estimates IQ. The former instrument was used to provide a profile of the subjects, while the latter instrument was used as one of the variables in examining the educational characteristics of subjects, along with mean overall grade point average and mean hours of ethics/philosophy. Since the demographic and IQ variables were not incorporated into a study purpose, their sudden appearance was confusing.

Gaul (1987) used the Judgment About Nursing Decisions (JAND) instrument to measure the dependent variables of nature of ethical choice and type of ethical action. The current JAND consists of six stories (in contrast to seven in the original tool) involving ethics in everyday nursing practice. Subjects are asked to respond both to (a) whether or not the nurse involved in the dilemma should engage in a predetermined list of five to seven actions and (b) whether or not the nurse involved in the dilemma is realistically likely to participate in these actions. The predetermined actions were determined by a nationally recognized panel of nursing ethics experts who rated each action according to the degree it conformed with behaviors advocated in the ANA *Code for Nurses.* Gaul noted that validity and reliability were well-established for the JAND but, with one exception, did not present these data. She could have strengthened her study and added to the body of knowledge about the JAND by conducting validity and reliability testing with her sample. In addition to the JAND instrument, Gaul also used a demographic work sheet.

Data Analysis, Results, and Conclusions

Felton and Parsons study.   In the Felton and Parsons (1987) study, which focused on the effect of baccalaureate nursing students and of master's nursing students' formal education on ethical/moral decision making, data were analyzed using *t* tests. Although two groups, such as the preceding ones, are appropriate for a *t* test, responses to the DIT are composed of nominal categories (i.e., should, should not, can't decide). Therefore, we questioned why the DIT's developer translated these categories into scores rather than frequencies. Despite this limitation, which was not noted by Felton and Parsons, results and conclusions for their two hypotheses related to the DIT were as follows: (a) master's nursing students scored significantly higher than baccalaureate nursing students on ethical/moral reasoning ($t = 3.00$, $p = .002$) and (b) master's nursing students did not differ significantly from baccalaureate nursing students on the number of ethical dilemmas resolved ($t = 1.53$, $p > .05$). From these results, Felton and Parsons concluded that formal education had a positive impact on ethical/moral reasoning but did not affect number of ethical dilemmas resolved. Typically, causal type relationships are not attributed to ex post facto designs. They also reported no significant correlation between levels of ethical/moral reasoning and dilemma resolution. Although this finding was interesting, it was not stated as a study hypothesis.

The third hypothesis, that master's nursing students would differ from baccalaureate nursing students in their attribution of responsibility, was not supported ($t = .02$, $p > .05$). The higher level of attribution of responsibility—justification—was rarely considered by either baccalaureate or master's students. Felton and Parsons concluded that ethical/moral reasoning was higher for the graduate students than for the undergraduate students in their study. They also seemed to infer that students did not know how to recognize ethical dilemmas or how to respond in a principled manner; these inferences did not seem to address their research hypotheses. The investigators' concern that nurses do not respond to ethical dilemmas in a principled way is understandable in light of recent research that suggests women justify moral decisions differently from men and that principles are not at the core of women's moral thinking. Although the typical female and male approach to justifying moral decisions appears to be different, we do not consider one approach superior to another as long as strong moral justification is given.

Gaul study.   Gaul (1987) also used t tests, but in conjunction with the Pearson correlation coefficient, to address her research questions. Results regarding her question of whether baccalaureate nursing students who have completed a nursing ethics course differ on ethical choice and on ethical action from baccalaureate nursing students who have not completed a course in nursing ethics were that there was no statistically significant difference on either choice ($t = -1.39, p = .17$) or action ($t = -1.57, p = .12$). However, Gaul observed that the group who had taken the ethics course did have a higher mean score on both choice and action than did the control group. Although the difference in means was not statistically significant, it suggests that further study is indicated, perhaps with a larger sample size.

Gaul (1987) also raised the question of whether or not a significant relationship existed between ethical choice and ethical action in the students who took an ethics course and those who did not. Using the Pearson correlation coefficient, the control group showed a nonsignificant correlation between choice and action ($r = -.32$, $p = .34$); however, the experimental group showed a significant positive correlation between choice and action ($r = .87$, $p < .001$). Unfortunately, the article contained a typographical error concerning the preceding results that could mislead the reader. Gaul concluded that the strong relationship between ethical choice and ethical action in the experimental group lent support to the need for an ethics course in baccalaureate curriculums. This conclusion appeared somewhat tenuous in light of the total results. Although in her discussion Gaul returned to her conceptual framework of the ANA *Code for Nurses* to help explain her results, she never mentioned her second conceptual framework—Kohlberg's theory.

Frisch study.   Frisch (1987), in her study of value analysis as a method for promoting moral development of nursing students, first presented gain scores from pretest to posttest. Some researchers would question the technique of analyzing pretest-posttest gain scores rather than posttest scores across experimental and control groups. She then calculated an analysis of variance on repeated measures using the DIT P score for the pretest and posttest measures. She found that no statistically significant differences occurred.

However, the experimental group, although initially treated as one group, was actually composed of three clinical sections that Frisch (1987) noted did not have identical experiences. Data analysis was difficult to interpret at this point, but it appeared that gain scores for each of the three sections were used and that Section 02 showed a statistically significant difference ($F = 5.50$, $p = .05$). Frisch explained this result as follows: It was an historical factor of Section 02's direct involvement with an ethical problem that caused them personal discomfort that led to outside-of-class discussions with peers. We believe this datum suggests that the preceding experience may have caused a more powerful treatment effect regarding moral development than the value analysis technique.

In contrast to the DIT P scores discussed by Frisch (1987), the DIT stage scores were evaluated differently. Because the six stages of Kohlberg's moral development are ranked, the Wilcoxin sign rank test for ordinal data was used. Frisch found a statistically significant difference in stage score gain in the experimental but not in the control group. Her conclusion was that higher stage thinking (i.e., Stage 4, which focuses on a duty orientation, and Stage 5, which focuses on a contractual orientation) occurred in the experimental but not in the control group. Frisch offered an explanation for this result that supported the value analysis strategy. Viable alternative explanations not supporting the result would have strengthened her discussion.

Regarding *both* the DIT P score results and the DIT stage score results, Frisch (1987) concluded that the value analysis instructional strategy produced measurable change in the level of moral judgment of some students. Regarding the DIT stage scores, the conclusion may be valid; however, regarding the DIT P scores, the conclusion is questionable as other than the value analysis approach appeared to have caused the statistically significant difference in Section 02 of the experimental group.

Mustapha and Seybert study.   Finally, in the Mustapha and Seybert (1989) study, which assessed moral reasoning in one group of undergraduate nursing students and two groups of undergraduate liberal arts students, data were analyzed according to the Demographic Data Questionnaire, the Shipley

Institute of Living Scale, and the P and D scores of the DIT. Data related to demographic variables (e.g., marital status, annual family income, academic major, years of formal education, age, IQ, mean overall GPA, and mean hours of ethics/ philosophy) showed no statistically significant differences using separate analysis of variance (ANOVA) on each variable.

Regarding the P score (level of principled reasoning) and the D score (preference for principled reasoning over conventional or postconventional reasoning), results of a multivariate analysis of variance (MANOVA) showed no significant main or interactive effects for academic class. However, statistically significant main effects occurred both for group and for gender on the DIT P and D scores. To determine where the difference occurred among the three groups on the variables of group and gender, ANOVA procedures were performed separately on the P and D scores. Results showed significant differences for gender and group on the P score but not the D score of the DIT.

Results regarding gender were as follows: Regarding the DIT P score, a main effect for gender occurred ($F = 5.83$, $p < .05$), leading to the conclusion that females had significantly higher DIT P scores than did males. This finding does not support some of the literature about gender differences; that is, that males tend to score higher on principled reasoning than do females. Mustapha and Seybert (1987) did not discuss reasons why women in their study scored higher on principled reasoning than did men. Were their IQ's higher? Did they take more hours of ethics/philosophy?

Results regarding group were as follows: The liberal arts students enrolled in the Foundations for the Future integrated curriculum had significantly higher DIT P scores than did the nursing group enrolled in the traditional curriculum ($t = 1.71$, $p < .05$). However, the nursing group enrolled in the traditional curriculum had significantly higher DIT P scores than the liberal arts students enrolled in the traditional curriculum ($t = 1.68$, $p < .05$). Mustapha and Seybert attributed this outcome to the nature of the nursing curriculum in that an ethics course was required for all nursing students. We wondered why this powerful variable was not controlled for at the beginning of the study. We also wondered what the rationale was for the use of t tests for planned comparisons, when the possibility of a t value being significant only by chance is increased with multiple t tests. We also wondered why ANOVA was used for gender and t tests for group.

Overall, Mustapha and Seybert (1989) concluded that integrated curriculums (like the Foundations for the Future curriculum described in their article) may facilitate higher levels of moral reasoning than traditional curriculums that include discrete liberal arts courses. The qualifier of "may" is justified by the design and data, as no nursing students were randomly assigned or enrolled in the integrated Foundations for the Future curriculum. Nowhere in their discussion did Mustapha and Seybert discuss or explain either their results in terms of Kohlberg's framework (and its operationalization through the DIT) or the strengths and limitations of their conceptualization.

Summary and Discussion

Taken together, these four ex post facto, pre- or quasi-experimental studies on the effects of ethics instruction on nursing students' moral development suggest the following:

1. Dissemination and timing of publication of these studies were not diverse; all studies were published from 1987 through 1989 in the *Journal of Nursing Education*. Although this is an appropriate vehicle for these studies, other avenues also exist.

2. In addition, several of the studies appeared to be outcomes of doctoral dissertations. This datum suggests that established investigators are not doing research on the topic and one must ask why ethical behaviors are professed to be valued in nursing education and yet

interventions to promote them are not being studied by senior researchers.

3. Kohlberg's theory of moral development was discussed in all four studies. At times Kohlberg's more recent works were not included, and the researchers varied in their ability to apply the theory throughout the study and to note limitations of the theory.

4. Although all four studies used comparison or control groups, the independent variable across studies varied sufficiently enough so that generalizability across studies would be difficult, thus impeding implementation into educational practice. In addition, all research was done at the baccalaureate and/or master's level, also impeding generalizability to other nursing students.

5. A clear picture of sampling procedures was difficult to determine in all four studies.

6. Unlike the variation in the independent variable, there was remarkable consistency in one of the instruments that measured the dependent variable. All of the studies except one used various parts of the Defining Issues Test. The one exception was Gaul's study; she used the Judgment about Nursing Decisions instrument.

7. Regarding analysis of data, typical statistics for interval data (e.g., *t* tests, ANOVA, MANOVA, Pearson correlation coefficients) were used, although at times the dependent variable appeared to represent other than interval data.

8. Finally, although variations and inconsistencies occurred, there appeared to be a beginning trend that instructional or curricular strategies that focus on ethics positively affect students' moral development or behavior.

To provide a solid basis for the teaching of ethics, we believe that more studies should be conducted on the effects of ethics instruction on nursing students' ethical awareness. However, experienced researchers, working in teams including junior researchers, should spearhead these studies and tighten the methodology. This tightening should include: (a) use of conceptual frameworks that are based on current research knowledge about women's moral development and behavior; (b) use of criterion measures that are an outgrowth of the preceding current conceptual frameworks on ethics; (c) use of consistency in and statement of rationales for determining sample size, sample characteristics, and study settings; (d) whenever possible, use of true experimental designs rather than ex post facto, pre- or quasi-experimental designs; (e) formulation of experimental treatments that are powerful enough to effect change; (f) justification for levels of measurement in data analysis; and (g) dissemination of results to a wider audience through such mechanisms as publication in a variety of appropriate journals, including research journals.

If most of the preceding suggestions are followed, the result would be a clearer and more consistent picture of the effects of ethics instruction on students. As a result of such efforts, we anticipate that generalizability, credibility, and, ultimately, applicability of results to nursing education practice would be enhanced.

PROCESS OF ETHICAL DECISION MAKING

We located two published studies (Pinch, 1985; Swider, McElmurry, & Yarling, 1985) that (a) focused totally or in part on student nurses and the process of ethical decision making and (b) were not primarily attitude or value studies. That part of the Pinch study that focused on attitudes is discussed in Part III of the monograph. In addition, other studies that included student nurses and ethical decision making but focused on attitudes or values are found in Part III and Part IV of the monograph, respectively.

Conceptualization

Pinch (1985) used Murphy's model as the basis for four (of five) research purposes that focused on ethical decision making. Murphy, basing her research on that of Kohlberg's, identified and categorized three models of nurse-patient relationships: (a) patient advocate model, (b) bureaucratic model, and (c) physician advocate model. Although Pinch noted Gilligan's work in relation to her fifth research purpose on attitudes (see Part III), she did not note it in the preceding models related to ethical decision making and nurse-patient relationships. This is a limitation of the study, as Gilligan disputed some of Kohlberg's findings on moral development.

Swider, McElmurry, and Yarling (1985) did not state a specific conceptual or theoretical framework for their study. Instead, they did a thorough review of the literature that focused on expository articles and research related to ethical decisions and social organizations, moral development, and nurses' roles and responsibilities. From this review of the literature, they identified a significant gap: the problem of ethical decision making and institutional constraints. This problem served as the basis for their research purposes.

Purpose

Regarding ethical decision making, Pinch (1985) identified four research purposes related to baccalaureate nursing students and graduated nurses: to determine respondents' (a) reactions to ethical dilemmas when ranking the three Murphy models, (b) degree of risk taking regarding the implementation of decisions involving ethical dilemmas, (c) assessment of institutional restrictions regarding the implementation of decisions involving ethical dilemmas, and (d) anxiety levels when involved with hypothetical ethical dilemmas. Since the investigator's overall purpose dealt with ethical *decision making,* some of the preceding purposes fit this objective better than others.

Swider, McElmurry, and Yarling's (1985) research purposes were difficult to discern. At one point in their literature review, they raised three questions that appeared to be the research purposes; however, in the next paragraph, they described two objectives of their study that also appeared to be the research purposes. Then in the last paragraph, under the heading entitled "significance," they raised three research questions. None of the three preceding approaches was totally consistent with one another. We identified their research purposes from the preceding three options by looking at the results and working from results back to purpose.

We determined that the following two objectives best met the purpose of the study: (a) to determine baccalaureate nursing students' decisions in response to a hypothetical nursing practice ethical dilemma and (b) to determine common themes or priorities among the students' decisions.

Methods

Design.   Pinch (1985) used a descriptive design that involved a questionnaire; one part included four hypothetical ethical dilemmas involving "No Code" orders, informed consent, confidentiality, and seemingly truthtelling. Swider, McElmurry, and Yarling (1985) used a descriptive design involving one case presentation about an ethical dilemma that involved a nurse's discovery of a patient's death due to a serious medication error by a resident and the resultant cover-up by the attending physician.

Sample.   In the Pinch (1985) study, the samples were drawn from students enrolled in selected NLN accredited baccalaureate nursing programs (109 freshmen and 103 seniors) and from 84 graduates (three to four years postgraduation). Other than their years postgraduate, no mention was made of any other characteristics of the graduates. The investigator obtained nursing students' volunteer responses by on-site testing at the selected nursing programs and by mailed questionnaires from the graduated respondents. However, Pinch did not make clear the sampling method or the criteria used for the selection of (a) the NLN nursing programs, (b) the inclusion of freshmen and seniors only, and (c) the postgraduation years of the graduates. In addition, the populations from which the samples were drawn were not discussed, and the return rate for that part of the sample who received the mailed questionnaire was only 21%, calling into question the validity of the results regarding the graduates.

In the Swider, McElmurry, and Yarling (1985) study, both a population and sample were included. The population

consisted of senior nursing students in baccalaureate programs in the midwest offering both undergraduate and graduate studies. From a list of the 35 graduate nursing programs
in the population, the investigators used random selection to
determine the first 20 schools for inclusion in the study. If a
school refused participation, it was replaced until the list
was exhausted. The investigators did not offer a rationale for
inclusion of the 35 graduate nursing programs when the
sample was senior baccalaureate nursing students, nor did
they explain the final data-generating sample of 16 schools
of nursing. From these 16 schools, with permission of each
dean from each school, a total of 146 small groups containing 755 students emerged. Each school had a mean of 9
groups, with a mean of 5 students per group. Generic students formed the vast majority.

Instruments.   Pinch (1985) used a three-part questionnaire that included the following: (a) the four previously
noted dilemmas that involved ethical decision making,
(b) a shortened form of the Pankratz Nursing Autonomy and
Patients' Rights Scale (see Part III regarding attitudes),
and (c) a demographic data profile. The four dilemmas were
developed by Pinch and were based on a review of relevant
literature. The decision making for each dilemma involved
the four research purposes (i.e., rank ordering of models, degree of risk taking, degree of institutional restrictions, and
anxiety levels). With the exception of the rank-ordering purpose, subjects responded to Likert-type scales to address the
other research purposes. In addressing content validity, Pinch
could have strengthened the development of the hypothetical
dilemmas by use of outside experts in addition to the literature review. Also, to establish interrater reliability, Pinch
could have established criteria for case construction; each
case then could have been assessed by reviewers to determine
whether, and to what degree, the criteria were met.
   In the Swider, McElmurry, and Yarling (1985) study, the
investigators defined the hypothetical case they developed as

a "a descriptive statement of situational factors" (p. 109). The case was reviewed and critiqued by registered nurses, a philosopher, a lawyer, and a nursing administrator. However, the nature and outcome of the review and critique were not discussed by the investigators. A strength of the study was that the investigators did develop the following criteria for the case: (a) negligence by a health provider, (b) maximum injury to a patient, (c) enhancement of the social identification of the nurse with the family, (d) clinical realism, (e) accuracy of detail, (f) appropriate length, and (g) intelligibility. Swider, McElmurry, and Yarling did not clearly specify who verified the validity or reliability of the criteria or how the criteria were applied to the case. Based on the criteria, our review of the case (which is presented in its entirety in the article), was as follows: that all of the predetermined criteria for the case were met, with the exception of length (over 600 words). The case presentation could have been shortened by eliminating some background details not pertinent to the ethical dilemma.

Data Analysis, Results, and Conclusions

Pinch study. In the Pinch (1985) study, data were analyzed appropriately using percents, median scores, and chi-square analysis. Major results were as follows: (a) regarding types of nurse-patient relationship models, a statistically significant difference occurred between the freshman group and the senior and graduate groups (chi square = 42.5, $p < .01$); (b) regarding high versus low risk taking, a statistically significant difference occurred between the freshman group and the senior and graduate groups (chi square = 18.93, $p < .01$); (c) regarding high versus low institutional restrictions, a statistically significant difference occurred between the freshman and senior groups and the graduate group (chi square = 10.1, $p < .01$), and (d) regarding high versus low anxiety about ethical dilemmas, a statistically significant difference occurred between the freshman and senior groups and the graduate group (chi square = 12.35, $p < .01$). A limitation of the results was that they were presented in a way that was difficult to follow.

Based on the preceding results, Pinch (1985) lumped conclusions together in the body of the article, but tended to discuss the dependent variables as pairs in the abstract. The abstract conclusions were as follows: (a) freshmen were less likely to select the patient advocate model and to take risks and (b) graduates' perceptions of restrictions and of anxiety were lower than the student groups. Conclusion *a* preceding could have been strengthened by noting the two other comparison models, by stating the levels of risk, and by noting that freshmen were being compared against seniors and graduates. Conclusion *b* preceding could have been strengthened by designating the levels of restrictions and anxiety, and by noting that the graduates were being compared against freshman and seniors.

In the discussion, Pinch (1985) briefly discussed Kohlberg, but never explicitly mentioned Murphy, whose three models served as the conceptual basis for the first research purpose. However, Pinch did offer some plausible explanations for the results and also noted that the results should be read cautiously. We agree with this assessment because of lack of clarity about sample characteristics and because of the low return rate (21%) of the questionnaire for the graduates. The latter point raises questions about the characteristics of the graduates who did respond and the generalizability of the study results.

Swider, McElmurry, and Yarling study. In the Swider, McElmurry, and Yarling (1985) study, data were analyzed appropriately using frequency counts, percents, mean scores, and chi-square analysis. In addition, to classify student decisions, the following three categories derived from the nursing literature were used: (a) patient-centered decisions, (b) physician-centered decisions, and (c) bureaucratic-centered decisions. Content analysis was used to place students' written decisions into categories and then frequencies per various categories were tabulated. The investigators did not note whether validity and reliability of the content analysis was done or, if done, the results of this process.

Major results were as follows: (a) from the 16 schools, the 146 small groups made a total of 1,163 decisions (mean of 8 per group) in their attempts to resolve the ethical dilemma in the hypothetical cover-up case; and (b) of all the decisions made, 105 were patient-centered, 221 were physician-centered, 698 were bureaucracy-centered, and 139 were designated as "other" as they did not fit the three preceding categories. Other results included a total of 107 decisions from written minority reports, the majority of which was classified as bureaucracy-centered.

As part of the procedure, each group was asked to read the case and determine in writing what action the group would take to resolve the ethical dilemma. They were then asked to assume that the preceding action was unsuccessful and determine in writing what the next action of the nurse should be. The preceding procedure continued until the group perceived that the nurse had exhausted all reasonable actions. The first and last decisions of the groups were then analyzed.

First decisions of the groups tended to be categorized as bureaucracy-centered (89%), physician-centered (8%), and other (3%); last decisions of the groups tended to be categorized as patient-centered (29%), bureaucracy-centered (27%), physician-centered (14%), and other (29%). The last decision total as reported in the article added up to 99% and not 100%. The investigators performed further analysis on type of student (generic students or RN students), type of degree (baccalaureate educational degree or other), prior experience with an ethical dilemma in practice similar to the hypothetical case (yes or no), and prior clinical experience (yes or no). Although chi-square analysis was useful and showed that there were no significant differences in group decisions based on the preceding characteristics, analysis of these subgroup characteristics was not stated as a research purpose.

Regarding the two stated research purposes, the investigators reported the following conclusions (conclusion *a* was explicitly stated by the investigators; conclusion *b* was inferred by the monograph authors based on the commentary in the discussion): (a) senior nursing baccalaureate students were confused and unclear about the endpoint of nurses' responsibilities in the ethical dilemma case presented to them and (b) a fourth category (collective-action centered) should be added to the existing three categories (patient-centered, physician-centered, bureaucratic-centered). The investigators then commented that these four major categories and their subcategories could be used to describe nursing students' decisions regarding hypothetical ethical dilemmas in nursing practice. The preceding conclusions were congruent with the results of the analysis of the data, but they did not answer precisely the research objectives as stated in the article. However, the investigators did discuss implications of their study for research and practice and also stated recommendations for further study.

Summary and Discussion

Taken together, these two studies on ethical decision making suggest the following:

1. The use of conceptual or theoretical frameworks was inconsistent, with one study having an explicit framework designated, and the second study inferring the possibility of a framework. The investigators of both studies were not consistent in use of the framework throughout the study.

2. The investigators of both studies stated research purposes, although in one study the purposes were clear and in the second study the purposes were ambiguous.

3. Descriptive methods were common to the two studies.

4. Sampling procedures were not clear in either study, and rationales for sampling decisions were omitted.

5. Both validity and reliability measures of the instruments could have been strengthened in both studies.

6. Both studies used appropriate data analysis techniques.

7. The conclusions of both studies were not clearly articulated.

8. Both studies were limited by the use of hypothetical, investigator-developed ethical dilemmas.

9. Despite the limitations of both studies, they added valuable baseline data to nursing science about the process of ethical decision making.

Although ethical decision making in nursing practice is important because of the frequency with which nurses face ethical dilemmas, we found it surprising that only two educational studies primarily involving nursing students focused on this process. Both studies were published in 1985, and we wondered why no further published research studying this phenomenon has occurred over the past six years. Perhaps lack of funding for educational research and ethics could be a factor.

The results and conclusions of both studies, although somewhat flawed, give pause for thought. Ethical decision making appeared to be a process that nursing students felt uncomfortable with and confused about in their roles, in their task responsibilities, and in their decisions. Certainly, such states of discomfort and confusion have implications for nurse educators and the overall curriculums they develop. Systematic curricular efforts are needed to ensure that students develop the knowledge base and experiences they need to feel more self-confident about ethical decision making in clinical practice.

UNETHICAL STUDENT AND FACULTY BEHAVIORS

We located five studies on unethical student and/or faculty behavior. Carmack's (1984) study focused on student plagiarism. Hilbert (1985, 1987, 1988) authored three of the five studies, which built on one another and focused on unethical student behaviors, whereas Theis (1988) focused on students' perceptions of unethical teaching behaviors of faculty.

Conceptualization

Carmack (1984) reported she could find no literature to guide her research, whereas in Hilbert's first two studies (1985, 1987), the literature on academic fraud was reviewed and reported, although no explicit conceptual framework was identified. However, in Hilbert's 1988 study, while using Kohlberg's framework as a basis for the hypotheses on moral development and nursing students' unethical behaviors, Hilbert did not note any limitations of Kohlberg's theory as a framework for the study.

Theis (1988), in looking at unethical teaching behaviors of faculty, appropriately reviewed the literature and noted an important gap on this topic. Consequently, her study focused on this gap and was conceptualized using Statement II of the American Association of University Professors' *Statement on Professional Ethics* that highlights the moral principles of respect for persons, beneficence, and justice. Although these principles are widely known and used, the conceptualization would have been strengthened by relating them to the American Nurses' Association's current *Code for Nurses* rather than solely from a related discipline's code.

Purpose

Although not stated as purposes of her study, Carmack (1984) raised four significant questions related to (a) faculty members' perceptions of the frequency of student plagiarism, (b) how faculty members handle plagiarism, (c) what factors contribute to faculty members' actions in managing plagiarism, and (d) the effectiveness of methods used by faculty members to resolve plagiarism.

Hilbert's 1985 article focused in part on the following: (a) the incidence of senior nursing students' unethical behaviors in both classroom and clinical settings; (b) the relationship between unethical behaviors in these two settings; and (c) the relationship between age, sex, and transfer status on unethical student behaviors. In the 1987 publication, Hilbert replicated the purpose in letters *a* and *b* preceding but with a larger and more diverse group of students. Hilbert also replicated the variables of age and sex noted in letter *c* preceding but added grade point average and ethnicity. A shift in purpose was to compare the incidence of unethical classroom behaviors for nursing and non-nursing students at the same schools and to determine students' reasons for their unethical behaviors. In the third publication, using Kohlberg's framework, Hilbert (1988) again shifted focus and looked at the relationship between level of moral judgment and the incidence of unethical classroom and clinical behaviors in upper division nursing students. Hilbert's three studies were derived appropriately from a gap identified in the literature, and the research questions/hypothesis were clearly stated.

In her study, Theis (1988) clearly stated her purpose: to design an instrument that would allow nursing students to identify their perceptions of unethical teaching behaviors of faculty. She then went on to conceptually define unethical teaching behaviors; however, the definition was so broad that some meaning was lost.

Methods

Design. Carmack (1984) collected her descriptive data using personal interviews that were tape-recorded; she inferred that permission was obtained for the taping. Hilbert (1985, 1987, 1988) and Theis (1988) used survey research designs that involved subjects' responses to written questionnaires. These designs were appropriate due to the exploratory nature of the research and the research questions raised.

Sample. Carmack's (1984) nonprobability sample consisted of 21 faculty members from 11 different schools of nursing that included diploma, associate degree, baccalaureate, and graduate programs throughout the country. For each subgroup, the *n* was so small that we wondered why she selected this approach; she gave no rationale in the article.

All three of Hilbert's studies involved students, but the type and numbers varied. In the 1985 study, Hilbert's sample was comprised of 101 last-semester senior baccalaureate nursing students. Hilbert, however, did not specify the nature of the institution(s) these students represented. In contrast, in the 1987 study, Hilbert noted that the sample was comprised of (a) 210 senior nursing students from a total of four sites in Wisconsin, California, and Pennsylvania, and (b) 21 senior behavioral science students from one of the preceding sites to serve as a comparison group. In the final study, Hilbert (1988) included 63 of 290 (22%) upper division nursing students who agreed to participate in the study and who were matriculated in a private university in the mid-Atlantic region. Hilbert did not, however, note the low participation rate as a serious limitation of this study. In none of the studies did Hilbert give rationales for the number, type, or location of students chosen, nor was Hilbert consistent in reporting informed consent or target populations. These data would have clarified how Hilbert replicated and/or extended the reviewed studies.

Theis's (1988) sample was comprised of 204 senior baccalaureate nursing students who gave informed consent and who were located in three NLN accredited programs in the midwest. Like Hilbert, Theis did not give a rationale for number, type, or location of students chosen. In all four studies, it was difficult to determine the sample from the population.

Instruments. As previously noted, Carmack (1984) conducted personal, taped interviews of about one hour in length. Carmack did not give examples of interview questions nor did she address validity or reliability issues.

For all three of Hilbert's studies, the Hilbert Unethical Behavior Survey was used. This survey contains a listing of 11 unethical clinical and 11 unethical classroom behaviors. The latter behaviors were obtained from a previously used tool and both types of behaviors in the 1985 study were assumed to have content validity. Overall, coefficient alpha for the 22 items was .67. Actual validity, rather than assumed, would have strengthened the 1985 study. In addition, a coefficient alpha for each subpart of the instrument would have increased the investigator's insight into the survey's internal consistency. In the 1978 and 1988 studies, Hilbert strengthened the validity of the tool by noting that content validity was established and not assumed as in the 1985 study. For Hilbert's 1988 study on moral development and unethical behavior, the shortened version of the Defining Issues Test (DIT) was also used. Hilbert noted that over the years the DIT has been shown to have adequate validity and reliability; however, no specifics about the outcomes of this adequacy were reported.

Theis's (1988) purpose was to design an instrument that focused on unethical teaching behaviors as perceived by students. She used free response data to establish content validity; however, she noted no other mechanisms for obtaining content validity nor did she mention reliability.

Data Analysis, Results, and Conclusions

Carmack study. Carmack (1984) reported her results using descriptive statements and statistics. Half of the faculty members she interviewed thought plagiarism was common, but most of them believed it was due to nursing students' lack of knowledge about how to write papers. Although Carmack did not seem aware of this inconsistency from the preceding sentence, the most frequent incident of plagiarism she cited was students' making up home visits ($n = 6$). Although Carmack presents much interesting data, it was difficult to relate the data to the research questions. No explicit conclusions were stated, although Carmack did *imply* that faculty members have difficulty in imposing sanctions for plagiarism. However, this implied conclusion was not entirely consistent with the data as presented.

Hilbert studies. Hilbert (1985, 1987, 1988) used a variety of descriptive and inferential data analysis techniques to address the research questions; the majority of the results are reported here. In the 1985 study, using percentages and ranges, Hilbert reported the following results and conclusions: the classroom behaviors considered most unethical by students were taking an exam for another student (99% of students) and cheating on an exam (98% of students); the unethical classroom behavior most frequently engaged in by students (27%) was copying materials from sources without footnoting them in papers. The clinical behaviors considered most unethical by students were recording that treatments, medications, or observations were done when they were not (100% of students) and coming to clinical while under the influence of drugs (98% of students); the unethical clinical behavior most frequently engaged in by students (59%) was taking hospital equipment home. A series of *t* tests on the variables of gender and transfers led to one significant finding: females engaged in more unethical classroom behaviors than did males ($p = .027$). In addition, correlations for the variable of age tended to be statistically not significant. Hilbert used the Pearson correlation coefficient to determine the relationship between students who engaged in unethical classroom and unethical clinical behaviors. The result was significant ($r = .57, p < .001$), indicating a positive relationship between the two.

In the 1987 study, Hilbert again used percentages and ranges to determine the extent of students' involvement in unethical behavior. As in the earlier study, the most common unethical classroom behavior engaged in by students was copying and not footnoting source materials in papers (52% of students). However, the most common unethical clinical behavior engaged in by students shifted from taking hospital equipment home to discussing patients in public or with other than health care staff (73% of students). Regarding the latter, students felt the patients' anonymity was preserved and that they needed to discuss their concerns with others. As before, results showed a significant positive correlation between classroom and clinical dishonesty ($r = .57, p = .00000$). A strength of Hilbert's 1987 study was the comparison of data with the 1985 study, and the plausible explanations offered for differences in the results.

In Hilbert's 1987 study, when nursing and non-nursing students were compared using a *t* test, no significant differences emerged between the two groups. On the other hand, in contrast to the 1985 study, the 1987 study showed no significant difference in unethical classroom or clinical behaviors between men and women. Students stated that the most common reason for engaging in unethical classroom behaviors was pressure for good grades, and the most common reason for engaging in unethical clinical behaviors was lack of perception that the behavior was unethical.

In Hilbert's 1988 study related to moral development and unethical behavior, the Pearson correlation coefficient was used to test two hypotheses. The first hypothesis, that an inverse relationship existed between level of moral development and frequency of unethical behaviors in the classroom, was not supported. However, the second hypothesis, that an inverse relationship existed between level of moral development and frequency of unethical behaviors in the clinical area, was supported ($r = -.243$, $p = .027$). Hilbert discussed these results regarding moral development in terms of the conceptual framework—Kohlberg's theory. This discussion was a strength of the study, as was the discussion about plausible explanations for the contradictory results in the two hypotheses. These discussions *indirectly* suggested that Kohlberg's theory may not have best explained the study results. We agree with this suggestion as Hilbert's sample was predominately female (whereas Kohlberg's sample on stages of moral judgment was male). As with Hilbert's other studies, unethical clinical and classroom behaviors were significantly and positively correlated. The most common unethical classroom and clinical behaviors that students engaged in were the same ones noted in the 1987 study.

Theis study. Theis (1988), in describing unethical teaching behaviors as perceived by students, categorized her data using content analysis. This technique was appropriate for an exploratory study. However, the precise procedures of the content analysis and how validity, reliability, and mutually exclusive categories were obtained were not addressed. Likewise, operational definitions for the ethical principles of respect for persons, justice, and beneficence were omitted, although the incidents that emerged from the content analysis were classified according to one of these three principles. Theis reported her primary result as follows: students, in both classroom and clinical settings, perceived that faculty most frequently violated the ethical principle of respect for persons. Examples included ridicule and sarcasm regarding students (in the classroom) and invasion of privacy and lack of consent regarding patients (in the clinical setting).

Summary and Discussion

Taken together, these five studies on unethical student and/or faculty behaviors suggest the following:

1. The conceptual frameworks used (both Kohlberg's theory and an ethical principle approach) would be open to question today, especially when the sample is composed primarily of women.

2. These five studies were primarily exploratory in nature, with concomitant methodological problems centering mostly around validity and reliability issues.

3. Demographic factors and unethical behaviors appeared to have little relationship.

4. Both students and faculty were perceived to engage in unethical classroom and clinical behaviors.

5. A consistently positive and statistically significant relationship existed between unethical classroom and unethical clinical behaviors.

Overall, the investigators' conceptualizations of their studies suggest that Kohlberg's theory influenced them strongly. Yet, concerns about use of his theory for women have been reported for some time. Although Hilbert (1985, 1987, 1988) and Theis (1988) were sensitive to validity of their instruments, overall, gaps existed. Future investigators interested in this topic should be careful to fill and/or report gaps related to both validity and reliability. Since demographic factors appeared to have little or no relationship to unethical behaviors, both faculty and students should be cautious in stereotyping unethical behaviors based on such factors.

The study results also suggested that at times both faculty and students were unaware of their unethical behaviors. Both groups need to obtain more insight into their behaviors, perhaps through planned interventions that increase their knowledge about ethical behaviors. Of all the results, the following was the most consistent: students who exhibited unethical behaviors in the classroom also were most likely to exhibit unethical behaviors in the clinical setting. This result has strong implications for student guidance. These students may have to be counseled out of nursing programs, or be given considerable assistance in recognizing the short- and long-term consequences of unethical behavior on self, patients, and the profession.

With the integrative review and critique of Part II on "Research of Curriculums, Curricular Strategies, and Ethics" complete, we now address Part III on "Research on Attitudes of Nursing Students and Faculty toward Ethical Issues."

Part III

Research on Attitudes of Nursing Students and Faculty toward Ethical Issues

In this section of the monograph, we include research studies related to attitudes of nursing students and nursing faculty toward various ethical issues. The 14 studies reviewed are related to clinical contexts of a variety of faculty and nursing student experiences. The studies reviewed are discussed in four categories: attitudes related to abortion, attitudes related to acquired immunodeficiency syndrome (AIDS), attitudes related to aggressiveness of nursing care for terminally ill patients, and attitudes related to patients' rights.

ATTITUDES RELATED TO ABORTION

We included five published research reports related to nursing student attitudes toward abortion in this review (Elder, 1975; Fischer, 1979; Hurwitz & Eadie, 1977; Rosen, Werley, Ager, & Shea, 1974a, 1974b). One study (Rosen et al., 1974a) also measured attitudes of nursing faculty toward abortion. The two reports by Rosen et al. (1974a, 1974b) were different aspects of one study. Reports by Elder (1975) and Fischer (1979) each included two related studies.

Conceptualization

The 1973 United States Supreme Court decision to ease legal constraints on abortion served as a framework in three of the reports (Elder, 1975; Rosen et al., 1974a, 1974b), although the research by Rosen et al. (1974a, 1974b) was conducted in 1971, before the Supreme Court ruling. The investigators did not state a specific theoretical framework for their studies. Hurwitz and Eadie (1977) placed their innovative study related to students' dreams within a framework of developmental psychology, citing research and theories of Erikson, Freud, Adler, Jung, Piaget, Breger, and Shapiro.

69

The study by Hurwitz and Eadie (1977) was the only study of the five listed which did not specifically use the term *attitudes;* the dependent variable was conceptualized as "psychologic impact" of participation in abortion. Fischer (1979) stated that attitude toward abortion was conceptualized as a predisposition to respond favorably or unfavorably to issues concerning abortion. Although Elder (1975) and Rosen et al. (1974a, 1974b) did not state their specific conceptualizations of attitude toward abortion, general characteristics of these attitudes were described in terms of approval/disapproval and permissiveness/restrictiveness (Elder, 1975) and favorable/unfavorable attitudes toward abortion (Rosen et al., 1974a, 1974b).

Purpose

The purpose was clearly indicated for each of the studies. Rosen et al. (1974a) compared attitudes toward abortion of students and faculty in nursing, medicine, and social work, as well as attitudes of the general population. In presenting data from their larger study on family planning, Rosen et al. (1974b) focused on the relationship between type of educational program and nursing students' attitudes toward abortion. Their purpose was to identify organizational characteristics that facilitate preparation of students to meet the needs of abortion patients.

Elder (1975) identified the need to study the relationship between nursing students' attitudes toward the 1973 Supreme Court decision and the reasons students accept as justifying an abortion. Fischer (1979) stated two specific goals for his research: (a) to evaluate the separate effects of attitudinal and context variables on students' judgments of hypothetical abortion patients and (b) to examine abortion as a potential stigma in a woman's medical history.

Hurwitz and Eadie (1977) sought to determine the psychologic impact on nursing students of participation in abortion and other educational experiences. These investigators noted that a secondary aim was to identify some of the conflicts and fears underlying anxiety that nursing students experience in abortion situations.

Methods

Design. In view of the exploratory nature of these studies, the investigators' selection of survey research designs was appropriate. Rosen et al. (1974a, 1974b) and Elder (1975) used descriptive designs in which participants completed questionnaires measuring attitudes toward abortion issues. Fischer (1979) incorporated into the study design a random distribution of different combinations of a hypothetical situation within a 3 × 3 factorial design. The research design of Hurwitz and Eadie (1977) provided for investigation of psychologic impact of participation in abortion within the natural context of student learning. This design, however, in which the dependent variable was measured at four different time intervals, allowed for serious threats to internal validity; that is, uncontrolled variables related to student activities at various times of data collection may have affected measurement of outcomes.

Sample. No rationale was provided by any of the investigators for sample size. The largest study was that of Rosen et al. (1974a, 1974b) who, in a nationwide survey, implemented a careful plan for stratification by size of school, size of community, religious affiliation, and type of program and degree, including 6,333 student nurses in the final sample of 47 nursing schools.

Elder (1975) used a convenience sample of 167 nursing students for her first study. She stated that these subjects were drawn from associate degree, diploma, and baccalaureate programs, but did not specify the level of the students. In her second study, Elder sampled 264 senior nursing students from associate degree, diploma, and baccalaureate programs.

Fischer's (1979) study of student nurses included 198 in the first study and 156 in the second study. He did not provide specific information about level of the student or type of program, but did specify that three training hospitals were used for the first study, and two training hospitals were used for the second study.

Hurwitz and Eadie (1977) encountered difficulties in obtaining a stable sample of nursing students for their study. They drew their sample from a population of 63 nursing students in their first year of one upper-divisional program; however, the number of completed questionnaires varied for each of the four weeks of data collection, ranging from 30 to 47.

In the studies which reported demographic information related to gender and religion, females constituted 96% to 99% of the participants. In view of the anticipated influence of the Catholic religion on attitudes of students toward abortion, it is important to note the considerable variation in percentages of Catholic students in the various samples. In the studies by Rosen et al. (1974a, 1974b) 36% of sample participants were Catholic, whereas in Fischer's (1979) study Catholics comprised 62% of the first sample and 52% of the second sample. In Elder's second study (1975) 54% of the sample was Catholic. Catholic nursing faculty constituted 29% of the sample by Rosen et al. (1974a).

The first study by Elder (1975) did not provide information about gender or religion. Although Hurwitz and Eadie (1977) provided demographic data for the population from which the sample was drawn, this information was not reported for the sample.

Instruments.   With the exception of the study by Hurwitz and Eadie (1977), in which psychologic impact of participation in abortion was measured, instruments measured student attitudes toward abortion. The impact on attitudes of different profiles of women seeking an abortion was studied and incorporated such factors as number of children, reason for abortion, marital status, and the trimester of pregnancy in which an abortion was sought. The relationships of students' religious background and type of nursing education program to student attitudes toward abortion also were studied.

All of the studies employed some type of questionnaire or written survey. Rosen et al. (1974a, 1974b) stated that their questionnaire, a six-point modified Likert scale, had been pretested. The investigators provided no information about content validity of the instrument, but cited reports that dealt with related aspects of the survey. The instrument, designed to measure attitudes toward broad aspects of family planning, contained only seven attitudinal items directly related to abortion (Rosen et al., 1974a) and only three of these items provided the focus for the report by Rosen et al. (1974b).

In Fischer's (1979) study, students were asked to make judgments about variations of hypothetical case profiles. Likert and semantic differential scales were used for student responses. Internal reliability estimates for the first and second studies were .91 and .74, respectively, for the Likert scale, and .89 and .97, respectively, for the semantic differential scale. Six additional items were used as an index to rate students' general attitudes toward abortion. The investigators cited a study that established reliability and predictive validity of this index, but impact of the scale in the first study appeared limited, in that only 170 of the 198 participants completed the scale. No rationale was provided in the report for this variation.

In Fischer's (1979) second study, internal consistency for the six items on attitude toward abortion was stated as .92, but no details for arriving at the figure were provided. Although not specifically stated in the report, all 156 participants in this second study appeared to have completed the six-item index.

In the first study by Elder (1975), a question about appropriateness for a pregnant woman to obtain an abortion was followed by six items, for which response alternatives of "yes," "no," and "uncertain" were given. Elder reported results indicating that the items formed a Guttman scale with a coefficient of reproducibility of .96, and a coefficient of scalability of .89. Also, a five-point scale was used to measure student attitudes toward the 1973 Supreme Court decision; no information was provided in the report about validity or reliability of this tool.

For the second study (Elder, 1975), the tools were revised, but specific changes were not stated clearly. An option of responding to variable times of pregnancy in relation to appropriateness of the abortion was added to the tool, and the five-point scale measuring attitudes toward the Supreme Court decision was changed to a six-point scale to discourage selection of an "uncertain" category. No measures of validity or reliability for the adapted tool were reported.

Hurwitz and Eadie (1977) used questionnaires to elicit responses related to student nurses' dreams after caring for patients undergoing an abortion and after a variety of other student experiences. Both validity and reliability of the questionnaires appeared limited, in that with successive administration of the questionnaires, both content and method of administration varied. These investigators also collected data from dream reports written by the students. Inconsistent methods of collection of these reports suggested that anonymity, although stressed to the students, may have been compromised, in that reports were returned in class, in the mail, and handed directly to the nursing instructor. Also, some reports contained students' names.

Data Analysis, Results, and Conclusions

Rosen, Werley, Ager, and Shea studies.   In analyzing the seven attitudinal items on the questionnaire, Rosen et al. (1974a) found that the percentages of college-educated general public with favorable attitudes toward freely accessible abortion (71%) were considerably greater than those for nursing students (42%) and nursing faculty (49%). The investigators specified the .05 level of significance, but did not provide a detailed description of chi-square analysis in which differences between students and faculty in nursing, medicine, and social work were estimated, making interpretation of these relationships difficult. However, data indicated that the smallest proportion of those with favorable attitudes toward abortion generally was found among nursing professionals. The nursing faculty category was the only one with less than half of the responses positive for helping a client obtain a legal abortion. When analyzing data according to religious categories, of Catholic students, nursing students were the least receptive toward abortion.

Rosen et al. (1974b) reported results of the above study in terms of organizational correlates of nursing students' attitudes toward abortion. The investigators stated that they used a .001 level of significance for chi-square analysis because the large sample size resulted in statistical significance at the usual levels even when percentage differences between comparison groups were very small.

When analyzed by type of educational program, the investigators found significantly fewer diploma students were in favor of abortion on demand when compared to associate degree students (chi square = 53.29) and baccalaureate students (chi square = 48.97). Only 37% of diploma students considered abortion appropriate under these circumstances, while approximately half of the baccalaureate and associate degree students approved. School Catholicism appeared to be a more important factor than type of program for abortion attitudes of Catholic baccalaureate students, but type of program appeared more important for Protestants. The investigators concluded that general cultural norms override counterpressures from organizations or policies, and that organizational characteristics seem to become relevant only in areas of ambiguity or controversy.

Fischer studies. The report by Fischer (1979) included two separate studies. Results of data analysis of both studies were not presented in relation to research questions or hypotheses, making it difficult to sort out findings in relation to each study variable. Results of analysis of variance in the first study showed that judgments of the appropriateness of the client's decision for an abortion were influenced strongly by the rationale given for the abortion ($F = 22.21$, $p < .005$). The woman's health elicited more support than either financial hardship ($p < .01$) or job satisfaction ($p < .01$). Personal convictions of respondents also strongly influenced judgments of the case situation. A striking finding was that subjects generally opposed to abortion were more apt to deprecate the woman in the case study even when the pregnancy posed a serious threat to her health.

In the second study by Fischer (1979), analysis of variance indicated a strong main effect of the hypothetical woman's history on favorable evaluation of the hypothetical woman's character ($F = 13.52$, $p < .005$). Again, attitudes were found to affect judgments of an abortion client under all conditions; anti-abortion respondents judged the hypothetical woman more harshly. Character ratings were significantly more favorable if the woman were a psychiatric patient or had undergone emergency surgery than if she had sought an abortion ($p < .01$). Judgments related to abortion were significantly more positive if the woman were single than if married ($p < .01$).

In both studies reported by Fischer (1979), regular church attendance by the respondent, but not religious affiliation, correlated inversely with favorable impressions related to the hypothetical woman, especially by Catholic respondents. Fischer (1979) concluded that both attitudes and case circumstances were important influences on subjects' impressions of the abortion client. Even when the need for an abortion was more obvious, for example the woman's health was endangered, attitude had a very substantial effect on the subjects' judgments.

Elder studies.   The report by Elder (1975) included two separate studies. Data analysis indicated that students had a great deal of difficulty answering situation questions because the time in pregnancy was not specified. This time factor was incorporated into Elder's second study and results indicated that acceptance of abortion under different circumstances varied dramatically with the time of the pregnancy under consideration. Sixty-one percent of the students thought that a woman in the first trimester of pregnancy should be able to obtain a legal abortion for all six reasons, but only 5% approved of it in the third trimester for all six reasons.

Threat to health was the only reason for abortion during all three trimesters that was approved by three-fourths of the students. Rape was approved by only one-third as a reason for third trimester abortion.

Catholic students were found to be less permissive under every circumstance in each trimester, although definitions of the terms related to "more or less permissive" were not clear in the study. No significant differences were found in general orientation toward abortion between students in associate degree, diploma, and baccalaureate programs.

Willingness of the respondent to participate in abortion procedures varied dramatically with the reason for abortion, the stage of the pregnancy under consideration, and the religious orientation of the respondent. Personal or social reasons for abortion, late stages of pregnancy, and Catholic religion of the respondent were all factors decreasing willingness to participate. Although the investigator noted several important implications for nursing from her findings, these implications were related more to nursing service than nursing education.

Hurwitz and Eadie study. In their study, Hurwitz and Eadie (1977) used chi-square analysis for questionnaire data, as well as content analysis for dream reports. Although differences between weeks of various student activities in relation to average number of dreams recalled were not statistically significant at the .05 level (chi square = 7.36, $p < .06$), the differences did approach statistical significance.

Content analysis of dreams indicated that of the nine dream reports after the abortion experience, six contained abortion-related material, whereas no similar events occurred in dreams from other weeks. We agree with the investigators' recommended caution in interpreting this finding, since the investigators' reference to the abortion experience when describing the rationale for the study to the students may have increased the probability that subjects would remember and report their abortion-related dreams. However, even with the small sample and methodological problems in this study related to inconsistent data collection protocols, results indicated that abortion-related material was evidenced in dreams. These data suggest that further research in content analysis of dreams could provide important information related to psychologic impact on students of participation in abortion experiences.

Summary and Discussion

When considered together, these five studies on attitudes toward abortion suggest the following:

1. Studies did not consistently identify a conceptual framework for the question of attitudes toward abortion.

2. Studies primarily have been exploratory, have used written surveys with convenience samples in limited geographical areas, and have presented little evidence of extending previous research on the topic.

3. Instruments used to measure attitudes toward abortion differed between each investigator and sometimes lacked documentation of validity and reliability. Also, most instruments did not differentiate between individuals who have or have not previously participated in nursing care for an abortion client.

4. Nursing students and nursing faculty, at the time the studies were conducted, tended to be less favorable toward abortion than other health professionals.

5. A number of variables influenced nursing students' attitudes toward abortion, including variables related to the student, such as religion, and variables related to circumstances of the case, such as trimester of pregnancy or reason for abortion.

6. Although these studies all included nursing students and/or faculty in the sample, the investigators did not emphasize the implications of findings for nursing education programs.

Several concerns arise from review of these five studies. First, there is a considerable gap in recent studies related to nursing student and faculty attitudes toward abortion; considerable contextual changes have occurred in our society since these studies were undertaken. Second, there is a need for data on the correlation between attitudes and behaviors of nursing students in relation to caring for an abortion client. Finally, implications of the findings for structuring nursing education programs must be addressed.

In spite of the various conceptual and methodological problems found in this review of research on attitudes related to abortion, we believe that these studies address a critical area in relation to research on ethics in nursing education. Through more consistent conceptualization of the problem, increased effort to build research on previous studies, and careful attention to issues of validity and reliability in research designs, further research should continue to identify important issues in relation to student and faculty attitudes toward abortion.

ATTITUDES RELATED TO ACQUIRED IMMUNODEFICIENCY SYNDROME (AIDS)

We located three studies related to attitudes of nursing students toward AIDS (Lawrence & Lawrence, 1989; Wertz, Sorenson, Liebling, Kessler, & Heeren, 1987; Wiley, Heath, & Acklin, 1988). Two of these studies (Lawrence & Lawrence, 1989; Wertz et al., 1987) also focused on knowledge related to AIDS. The Wertz et al. study focused primarily on nursing service, rather than nursing education, but since nursing students were a small part of the sample for the study, we included it in our review of the research.

Conceptualization

No conceptual framework was presented for these studies. Wiley et al. (1988) discussed findings in relation to the document, "Statement regarding risk versus responsibility in providing nursing care," an interpretative statement issued by the American Nurses' Association Committee on Ethics in 1986.

Purpose

The purpose of the study by Wiley et al. (1988) was to identify attitudes toward nursing care of patients seropositive for human immunodeficiency virus (HIV), so that curricular changes necessitated by the increased incidence of AIDS could be implemented. The other two studies (Lawrence & Lawrence, 1989; Wertz et al., 1987) focused on knowledge and attitudes of respondents before and after educational programs, with Lawrence and Lawrence (1989) also comparing attitudes of nursing and nonnursing groups.

Methods

Design.   Lawrence and Lawrence (1989) appropriately described Phase I of their study as nonexperimental. They stated that Phase II of their study, which incorporated a pretest-posttest format, was quasi-experimental, but the lack of a control group indicated a pre-experimental design. The report of the study lacked important details related to the design, such as length of time between pretest and posttest. The investigators did not refer to the potential testing effects of the pretest on posttest scores.

Wertz et al. (1987) also used a pre-experimental, pretest-posttest design. The posttest was given immediately after the educational program, and a follow-up assessment was done one month after the program. The investigators stated that the pretest and posttest comprised different parts of the questionnaire, but did not clearly indicate differences in the two parts.

The descriptive study by Wiley et al. (1988) used a written questionnaire to survey nursing students' attitudes related to care of AIDS patients. The procedure for data collection was not clearly stated, although the response rate (32%) was provided.

Sample.   Convenience samples were used in all three studies. Only Wertz et al. (1987) provided a rationale for their convenience sample of 1,247 (a 90% response rate) drawn from 36 sites in Massachusetts, noting that the pressure for immediate education to meet hospitals' projected needs for patient care precluded selection of a random sample of providers or a control group. Only 5% of this sample of 1,247 health care providers were nursing students.

Lawrence and Lawrence (1989) failed to distinguish between the terms *sample* and *population,* stating that the study population consisted of 182 persons. Of this total, 50 were baccalaureate nursing students (the level of the program was not specified), 42 were non-nursing college students, 60 were registered nurses, and 30 were non-nurse adults. All subjects participated in Phase I of the study, but only 50 baccalaureate nursing students, 42 non-nursing college students, and eight registered nurses participated in Phase II. The investigators did not specifically state that these were the same respondents that participated in Phase I of the study, making interpretation of findings difficult.

In the study by Wiley et al. (1988), the sample, drawn from one nursing school, consisted of 47 graduate nursing students, 18 registered nurse/bachelor of science in nursing (RN/BSN) completion students, and 77 junior and senior undergraduate students. The large range of clinical nursing experience of students in the sample, 28 days to 28 years, limits the generalizability of findings from this sample.

Instruments. Instruments were apparently developed by the investigators for each study; Wertz et al. (1987) did not state the origin of the questionnaire. Only Lawrence and Lawrence (1989) provided information about validity and reliability for their instruments, which measured both knowledge and attitudes; these investigators established content validity through an unspecified number of nurse experts, and used Kuder-Richardson formula 21 to estimate internal consistency (coefficient ranged from .75 to .93). In some sections of the report, these investigators stated that the instrument measured dependent variables of attitudes and beliefs, but no distinction was made between these terms, and findings were reported primarily in terms of attitudes.

Wertz et al. (1987) used questionnaires designed to measure both knowledge and attitudes of participants. Subjects completed 55 items of the questionnaire before the educational program and 43 different items immediately after the program. The same questionnaire was mailed to a subset of the sample one month after the educational program to assess whether the program had more than a short-term effect on knowledge and attitudes of the participants.

Wiley et al. (1988) designed a 66-item questionnaire to measure students' perceptions of their risk of HIV exposure through clinical practice, as well as their attitudes toward selected issues regarding nursing care of HIV-seropositive patients.

Data Analysis, Results, and Conclusions

Lawrence and Lawrence study. It was not clear why Lawrence and Lawrence (1989) used both a series of individual *t* tests and analysis of variance to analyze the same sets of data. We will discuss only the results of the analysis of variance, since this test appears more appropriate for analysis of the multiple groups. The hypothesis that nursing students have more knowledge and more positive attitudes about AIDS than liberal arts college students was not supported. Correlation coefficients calculated to compare knowledge and attitude scores indicated significant positive correlations between knowledge and attitudes about AIDS ($p < .001$). However, the investigators' conclusion that the data provided concrete evidence that education does make a difference in knowledge and enhancing positive attitudes appeared to go beyond the data presented.

Phase II of the study was related to effects of an educational program on posttest scores. Findings supported the hypothesis that the educational program increased participants' knowledge and attitude scores about AIDS ($p < .001$ for nursing student group). Baccalaureate nursing students had the greatest increase in knowledge and attitude scores. The conclusion that nurse educators may be unnecessarily concerned about the negative impact of AIDS on student recruitment and retention, in that nursing students in the study had positive attitudes toward patients with AIDS, appeared to be unsubstantiated by the data presented. Nursing students surveyed in this study had already committed themselves to the nursing program and might be expected to have more positive attitudes than other students, yet mean attitude scores on the pretest for nursing students were lower (36.38) than scores for non-nursing students (38.19).

Wertz, Sorenson, Liebling, Kessler, and Heeren study. Data analysis by Wertz et al. (1987) was presented without specifying nursing students as a separate category. Thus, it is impossible to attribute findings specifically to nursing students. Overall findings indicated significant increases in accuracy of knowledge, as computed with the McNemar test, related to seven of fifteen modes of transmission of AIDS and seven of eleven means of infection control. Areas in which there were statistically significant increases of knowledge included immediate discarding of needles without recapping; use of gowns, masks, and double gloves; quarantine of patients' rooms; and use of shoe protectors.

Attitudes of participants after the educational program shifted in the desired direction on six of nine questions ($p < .001$). These questions related to participants' perceptions of sufficient knowledge to protect themselves from contracting AIDS, feelings of competence in caring for AIDS patients, preference to avoid caring for AIDS patients, comfort in interacting with the lover of an AIDS patient, perceptions that AIDS patients can have nonsexual social contacts, and perceptions that if they got AIDS, others would think them homosexuals.

Responses of the one-month follow-up survey were compared with the same subjects' pretest and posttest responses,

using the McNemar test. Although the level of statistical significance was not provided in the report, the investigators
noted that changes remained significant for knowledge about
six modes of transmission, knowledge about eight modes of
preventing transmission, and five attitudes, suggesting that
posttest changes in both knowledge and attitudes were, for
the most part, retained. The investigators concluded that educational programs can result in significant changes in both
knowledge and attitudes, but did not address educational programs for nursing students.

   Wiley, Heath, and Acklin study.   In their study, Wiley et al.
(1988) reported that responses of graduate nursing students, RN/BSN completion students, and junior and senior
undergraduate students did not differ at a significant level
($p = .05$) in regard to worry about exposure to HIV or use of
protective measures. The investigators, however, did not
specify which statistical analysis was carried out to arrive at
this finding. A weighted mean of 54% of the students felt that
nurses should be permitted to refuse assignment to HIV-
seropositive patients. Twenty-one percent of the graduate
students, 40% of the RN/BSN completion students, and 45%
of the undergraduate students stated that they would defi-
nitely or probably refuse to treat HIV-seropositive patients.
We agree with the investigators' recommendations of caution
against generalizing findings of this small study to other populations, and agree, too, with their suggestion that faculty
incorporate into nursing curriculum discussions of ethical
and moral issues relating to nursing care of HIV-seropositive
patients.

Summary and Discussion

These studies have limited generalizability, having been undertaken in limited geographical settings with small convenience samples of nursing students. They indicate, however,
the need for further research related to the following:

1. Clarification of how attitudes of nursing students toward HIV-seropositive patients might affect nursing care of these patients.

2. Systematic study of effects of educational programs on development of both knowledge and positive attitudes toward AIDS patients for nursing students.

In view of the many concerns voiced by health professionals about care of patients with AIDS, the lack of systematic study of this problem as it relates to nursing students and faculty is surprising. It is imperative that nursing students and faculty understand the factual, ethical, and moral issues involved in providing care for patients with AIDS. Future studies with larger, more diverse samples of students and the use of qualitative, as well as quantitative, data could enhance our understanding of nursing student attitudes related to AIDS.

ATTITUDES RELATED TO AGGRESSIVENESS OF NURSING CARE FOR TERMINALLY ILL PATIENTS

We located two studies related to student attitudes toward aggressiveness of nursing care for terminally ill patients. Winget, Kapp, and Yeaworth (1977) focused on health professionals' attitudes toward euthanasia. Shelley, Zahorchak, and Gambrill (1987) carried out three related studies dealing with attitudes toward aggressiveness of nursing care for older patients and those with do-not-resuscitate (DNR) orders. Since only their second study included nursing students, this study will be the focus for this review.

Conceptualization

Winget et al. (1977) discussed several theorists in relation to decision making in medical ethics, including Parsons and Skinner. They also discussed the concept of euthanasia within the framework of the statement adopted by the American Medical Association in 1973, in which "mercy killing" is seen as contrary to the standards of the medical profession. The investigators conceptualized conflicts arising from attitudes toward euthanasia as intrapersonal or interpersonal in nature, a distinction that was useful in understanding the rationale for the study. Intrapersonal conflicts may arise from an individual's struggle for cognitive balance or consistency in attitudes and beliefs; this struggle may be intensified by the process of socialization into a new professional role which involves learning new attitudes and beliefs. Interpersonal conflicts may exist when attitudes and beliefs of physicians or nurses conflict with each other, or with those of the patient, the family, or society at large.

Shelley et al. (1987) did not state a specific conceptual framework that guided their study. However, they placed their research within a careful review of literature of the concept of do-not-resuscitate. The review of literature also included studies focusing on nurses' attitudes toward DNR orders, care of dying patients, and negative euthanasia, but did not address specifically attitudes of nursing students in relation to these variables.

Purpose

Winget et al. (1977) described attitudes of health workers and college students toward euthanasia. They explored interpersonal and intrapersonal conflicts which might affect the decision-making process of individuals faced with issues of fighting for or maintaining life.

Shelley et al. (1987) stated the intent of extending the research of Lewandowski, Daly, McClish, Juknialis, and Youngner (1985), a prospective study comparing nursing care among intensive care unit patients with and without DNR orders. Shelley et al. stated their specific purpose as testing the main and interactive effects of age and DNR orders on attitudes toward aggressiveness of nursing care. Although not stated in their purpose, the effect of student type on attitudes toward aggressiveness of nursing care was also tested.

Methods

Design. The study by Winget et al. (1977) was designed as an exploratory study using a questionnaire to elicit responses from medical, nursing, and college students and practicing nurses and physicians about attitudes toward euthanasia. Shelley et al. (1987) used a carefully designed factorial approach with independent variables of age, DNR orders, and student type.

Sample. Winget et al. (1977) used a sample of medical students ($n = 200$), college students ($n = 75$), nursing students ($n = 177$), registered nurses ($n = 75$), and physicians ($n = 30$). The sample of nursing students included 108 first-year students and 69 senior students. The investigators did not provide details about how their sample was selected.

For their study of 183 nursing students, Shelley et al. (1987) used a sample of 115 volunteer senior baccalaureate and 68 graduate nursing students. Information was not presented in the report regarding rationale for sample size or number of nursing programs represented by this sample.

Instruments. Winget et al. (1977) used a questionnaire developed by an interdisciplinary research group as part of a larger study; the investigators cited a reference for further information about construction of the questionnaire. Only five of the 50 items on the questionnaire were related to attitudes toward euthanasia, and it was these five items that formed the basis for this study. No information was provided for content validity or reliability of the instrument.

Shelley et al. (1987) used an instrument consisting of four different versions of a vignette; half of the vignettes described the patient as 72 years and the other half as 28 years. Within each of these two age versions, half of the vignettes described the patient as having DNR orders, and the other half did not refer to DNR orders. In their first study, the investigators randomly assigned the four different vignettes to subjects for completion. For the second study, this random assignment to the different types of nursing students was not stated, but it was implied. All versions of the vignette were followed by the same 13-item, six-point Likert scale, designed to measure the dependent variable: attitudes toward aggressiveness of nursing care. Content validity of the instrument was established by a systematic process and internal consistency reliability with Cronbach's coefficient alpha was obtained (.81).

Data Analysis, Results, and Conclusions

Winget, Kapp, and Yeaworth study.   In this study (1977), Winget et al. used descriptive statistics and Duncan's multiple range test, with a confidence level of .01, to analyze data related to the five items on the questionnaire. In responding to the statement "No matter what my personal beliefs, in my role as a nursing professional I would fight to keep the patient alive," 69% of first-year nursing students agreed, as compared to 41% of senior nursing students. To the statement, "Some patients should be allowed to die without making heroic efforts to prolong their lives," 66% of first-year nursing students and 88% of senior nursing students expressed agreement. When Duncan's multiple-range test was used to compare mean scores on the euthanasia subscale for each of the seven groups, significant differences were found in attitudes toward euthanasia, specifically between first-year and senior nursing students. First-year nursing students, along with non-nursing college students, had the least accepting attitudes of all groups toward euthanasia.

When responses to the total questionnaire were analyzed to evaluate general issues related to the dying patient and his family, the senior nursing students were found to have the most understanding and emphatic (*sic*) responses. Practicing nurses and nursing students were the only groups for which attitudes toward euthanasia were not positively correlated with other attitudes toward dying patients.

The investigators speculated that these findings might indicate that women, especially nurses, have learned to tolerate more indecision and inconsistency in their attitudes than men. The investigators also applied sociological theory to interpretation of their findings, which would indicate that a longer socialization process would more likely result in internalization of attitudes associated with a role. Thus the shorter length of educational programs for nurses in comparison with those for physicians may mean that nurses are less likely than physicians to internalize a consistent set of attitudes to use in resolving clinical dilemmas posed by a dying patient.

Shelley, Zahorchak, and Gambrill study. In this study, Shelley et al. (1987), using analysis of variance, found significant main effects related to type of student ($F = 4.96$, $p < .03$) and DNR orders ($F = 28.27$, $p < .000$). Graduate nursing students agreed less strongly with aggressive approaches than senior students, and attitudes toward care were less aggressive for the patient with DNR orders. Significant main effects due to patient age were not found, in contrast to main effects found in the investigators' first study with staff nurses. In this study, however, there was a significant interaction effect ($F = 4.3$, $p < .04$) between patient age and DNR orders. Using the Tukey HSD test ($p < .01$), the investigators found that DNR orders resulted in less agreement with aggressive care for the older patient, but not for the younger patient. No effect of age differences was found among patients without DNR orders.

We agree with the investigators' caution in assuming that nurses would respond to actual clinical situations as they did to the vignettes. Their discussion of overall results unfortunately did not consistently differentiate findings obtained with nurses and student nurses, making interpretation difficult. Although their results did support findings of

Lewandowski et al. (1985), who described care of DNR and non-DNR patients in an actual clinical setting, that study did not include student nurses.

The finding by Shelley et al. (1987) that of all groups in the study, undergraduate students responded more aggressively under all conditions, was discussed in relation to the possibility that students' high idealism may change when students encounter the realities of clinical practice. An unstated implication of the study is that nurse educators should be concerned with assisting students to identify appropriate levels of aggressive care for DNR patients.

Summary and Discussion

The two studies reviewed in relation to attitudes toward aggressiveness of nursing care for terminally ill patients differed in conceptual bases for the studies, tools used to measure the dependent variable, level of nursing student surveyed, and important aspects of research design. Nevertheless, some important considerations arise from the studies:

1. Both intrapersonal and interpersonal conflicts appear to influence attitudes of nursing students/nurses toward aggressiveness of care for terminally ill patients.

2. At higher levels of education, nursing students appear to exhibit less aggressiveness of care for terminally ill patients than beginning students.

Within the broad perspective of participation in decision making in medical ethics, it is important to better understand how nursing students resolve intrapersonal and interpersonal conflicts related to euthanasia. Attitudes appear to change as individuals are socialized in professional roles, indicating that nurse educators should provide opportunities for students to begin to internalize attitudes toward aggressiveness of care for terminally ill patients. The differences in attitudes toward aggressiveness of nursing care by nursing students at different levels which were identified in these studies indicate a need not only to define more clearly these differing attitudes, but also to help students interpret the expectations of DNR orders. As noted by Lewandowski et al. (1985), overtreatment can cause undue patient suffering, financial burdens, and waste of health care resources.

ATTITUDES RELATED TO PATIENTS' RIGHTS

We reviewed four studies of students' attitudes related to general issues of patients' rights. These studies dealt with attitudes toward (a) nursing disclosure of information to patients (Davis & Jameton, 1987); (b) rights of hospitalized patients (Kurtzman, Block, & Steiner-Freud, 1985); and (c) nursing autonomy, patients' rights, and traditional role boundaries (Cassidy & Oddi, 1988; Pinch, 1985). In Part II of this monograph, we have already reviewed the Pinch (1985) study in relation to ethical dilemmas in nursing. In this section, we address aspects of that study related to attitudes toward nursing autonomy, patients' rights, and traditional role boundaries.

Conceptualization

Pinch (1985) placed her study within the framework of Murphy's identification of three nurse-patient relationship models: the patient advocate model (the autonomous model), the bureaucratic model, and the physician advocate model. These models were a result of Murphy's investigation of the levels of moral reasoning of nurse practitioners, which was based on Kohlberg's theory of moral development.

None of the other studies were organized around a conceptual framework. Two studies, however, (Davis & Jameton, 1987; Kurtzman et al., 1985) referred to the American Hospital Association's Patient's Bill of Rights as a focus within the study. This document outlines the rights of the patient for information disclosure from a physician. Davis and Jameton (1987) viewed this Bill of Rights as a symbol of paternalism, noting that hospitals have no power to grant patient rights, since these rights are vested in the patient.

Purpose

Pinch's (1985) stated purpose was to examine for three levels of professional nurses the perception of degree of professional nursing autonomy, including attitude toward nursing autonomy, promotion of patients' rights, and rejection of the traditional role. The term *professional nurses* was confusing, since two of the levels consisted of freshmen and senior nursing students.

Cassidy and Oddi (1988) stated the purpose of their study as the determination of differences in perceptions of ethical dilemmas in practice and attitudes toward autonomy among four groups of nursing students. Attitudes toward autonomy were viewed in the context of patient advocacy, patients' rights, and traditional nursing role limitations.

The purpose of Davis and Jameton's (1987) pilot study was to explore attitudes of senior nursing and fourth-year medical students toward the nurse's role in the disclosure of information to patients. The investigators pointed out the lack of clarity of the role of nurses in disclosure of information to patients.

Kurtzman et al. (1985) stated a similar purpose: to compare attitudes of first- and fourth-year nursing and medical students toward the rights of hospitalized patients. They also identified associations between attitudes and student variables of age, sex, and ethnic origin.

Methods

Design. All of the reviewed studies were descriptive, using questionnaires to measure attitudes of students.

Sample. Cassidy and Oddi (1988) stated that a random sample was selected, but did not provide details about the selection process. All of the other studies used convenience samples. Investigators did not provide a rationale for sample size.

Pinch (1985) stated that she included students from selected departments of nursing with an approved baccalaureate nursing program, but did not provide the number of nursing departments sampled. Her total sample was stated as 294, although if the stated 109 freshmen, 103 seniors, and 84 graduates were included, the actual total sample would be 296. It was not clearly stated whether the graduates used as subjects were enrolled in a graduate nursing program. The majority of students in the sample (62%) were Catholic, which Pinch noted posed certain limitations in data analysis and interpretation.

Cassidy and Oddi (1988) randomly selected 236 female nursing students from students enrolled in a master's, degree-completion, and generic baccalaureate program at a university and in an associate degree program of a community college. Information was not provided about the size of the student population from which the 236 names were drawn. A 55% return rate of questionnaires mailed to these students resulted in a study sample of 130 nursing students. Of these 130 students, 45 were master's students, 33 were degree-completion students, 29 were generic baccalaureate students, and 23 were associate degree students. Master's students had completed at least 15 hours of their 36-hour educational program. Both groups of baccalaureate students had completed at least 90 hours and the associate degree students were enrolled in their final semester of the program. Fifty students (38.4%) had completed a course in ethics, and 64 (49.2%) had completed a seminar dealing with ethics.

Students in the studies by Davis and Jameton (1987) and Kurtzman et al. (1985) were from one institution. The investigators of these latter two studies noted that groups of nursing and medical students included in the sample differed considerably in relation to age and sex, with more females and younger students represented by nursing.

The study sample of Davis and Jameton (1987) included 28 senior nursing students and 28 senior medical students at one health science center. The investigators did not specify procedures for selecting the sample. There were significantly more female nursing students (23) than female medical students (11) and significantly fewer male nursing students (5) than medical students (17) (chi square = 9.05, p = .0026).

Kurtzman et al. (1985) included in their sample of Israeli students 49 first-year and 24 fourth-year nursing students, and 97 first-year and 32 fourth-year medical students. The investigators stated that the study population included all first-year and fourth-year medical students present in class the day the questionnaire was administered. Only half of the fourth-year medical students participated in the study, as the other half had a clinical assignment. Since students were randomly assigned to clinical settings, however, the investigators assumed that participants were representative of the fourth-year medical class. The investigators did not discuss the population of nursing students or provide information about how the sample of nursing students was selected.

Instruments.   Both Pinch (1985) and Cassidy and Oddi (1988) used the Pankratz Nursing Autonomy and Patients' Rights Scale (NAPRS) to examine three separate attitudes: nursing autonomy and advocacy, patients' rights, and rejection of traditional role limitations. The five-point Likert-type scale included 47 items, with subjects responding in terms of agreement/disagreement. Investigators of both studies provided references for the scale, as well as information related to development and previous testing of the scale in relation to validity and reliability.

Cassidy and Oddi (1988) measured perceptions of ethical dilemmas in nursing practice with Judgments About Nursing Decisions (JAND), an instrument that describes six stories depicting nurses in ethical dilemmas. The JAND was developed around a theoretical framework derived from the ANA's *Code for Nurses*. The investigators presented information for prior determination of face validity, content validity, empirical validity, and discriminant validity of the instrument. They reported that Ketefian's prior determination of reliability for the instrument indicated that the part of the instrument related to idealistic behavior had coefficients that ranged from approximately .70 to .73 (Cronbach's alpha), and that the part of the instrument related to realistic behavior had lacked internal consistency.

Prior to completing analysis of data for this study, Cassidy and Oddi (1988) tested the reliability of both the JAND and the NAPRS and eliminated items that were unreliable. Coefficient alpha values were computed for the modified instruments, and intercorrelations were determined for the modified subscales of the JAND and the NAPRS. Low reliability was found for both the original and modified JAND subscales. Cassidy and Oddi noted limitations of the study instruments, in that both instruments were in an early stage of development and empirical validation, and that the removal of unreliable items from the instruments may have compromised content validity.

Neither of the other two studies (Davis and Jameton, 1987; Kurtzman et al., 1985) addressed issues of validity or reliability for the instruments. For the study by Davis and Jameton (1987), participants responded to a questionnaire designed to measure attitudes toward nursing disclosure of information to patients. The instrument involved five case studies, to which students responded by indicating what they thought were the best, second best, and worst responses for the nurse to give in the specific situation. No information was provided about how the questionnaires were administered.

Kurtzman et al. (1985) developed a four-point Likert scale questionnaire to determine attitudes of students toward the rights of hospitalized patients in six different areas. Some of the questionnaire items were adapted from the American Hospital Association's Patient's Bill of Rights. The questionnaire also measured attitudes toward adequacy of a blanket consent form used in the hospital and individual responsibility for protecting patients' rights.

Data Analysis, Results, and Conclusions

Pinch study. Pinch (1985) used chi-square analysis ($p < .01$) to analyze the Pankratz questionnaire. Freshmen scores on the scale differed significantly from both senior or graduate levels. Freshmen scored significantly lower than the other two groups on attitudes toward nursing autonomy (chi square = 95.2), promotion of patients' rights (chi square = 31.1), and rejection of the traditional role in nursing (chi square = 89.2). Pinch noted that freshmen students have not yet been initiated in relation to nursing theory/ knowledge and professional issues of concern, and have ideas of role fulfillment from family, school, and society, rather from the process of professional education.

Cassidy and Oddi study. Cassidy and Oddi (1988) found that mean scores of the associate degree group on patients' rights and rejection of traditional role limitations exceeded those of the other three student groups. Scores for autonomy were similar for associate degree and generic baccalaureate students. There were no significant differences among groups on subscales measuring perceptions of ethical decision making.

Using one-way analysis of variance, significant differences were found among groups on autonomy ($F = 20.93$, $p = .000$), patients' rights ($F = 3.14$, $p = .027$), and rejection of traditional role limitations ($F = 5.51$, $p = .001$). Results of the Scheffe post hoc test indicated that associate degree and generic baccalaureate students scored significantly higher on autonomy than the degree-completion and master's students ($p = .05$). Associate degree students scored significantly higher than master's students on rejection of traditional role limitations ($F = 51$, $p = .001$). No significant differences were found between groups on perceptions of idealistic and realistic moral behavior.

Students who had taken a course in ethics scored significantly higher on autonomy ($F = 6.89$, $p = .009$) and rejection of traditional role limitations ($F = 10.25$, $p = .001$). However, those students who had not attended a continuing education ethics seminar scored significantly higher on autonomy ($F = 19.38$, $p = .000$) than those who had attended an ethics seminar.

The investigators noted that only tentative conclusions related to the study could be made, since both instruments used in the study were at an early stage of development and validation, and the JAND was found to have unsatisfactory reliability for this study. They suggested that one explanation for the finding that students attending an ethics seminar scored lower than those who did attend the seminar may be that the seminar allowed only superficial expoloration of ethical issues. Another explanation could be that the two groups differed in initial attitudes toward autonomy.

The investigators suggested that discussion of ethical theories is most effective when accompanied by opportunities to apply the theories in practice situations. They also noted that the study raised questions about whether the outcomes of courses in nursing ethics may be related more to professional values than to perceptions of ethical dilemmas in patient care.

Davis and Jameton study.   With chi-square analysis, Davis and Jameton (1987) found a statistically significant difference between senior nursing students and fourth-year medical students on 20 of 87 items on the questionnaire ($p = .05$). For 15 of these items, nursing students showed greater support than medical students for an active nursing role in disclosure, informed consent, expressing professional opinions, and patients' decision making.

The investigators interpreted the strong nursing interest in disclosure in relation to nursing concern for patient autonomy and nursing concern for the autonomy of nurses as professionals. Another explanation might be that the medical students were reluctant to relinquish the "power" of their professional role. The investigators, noting the argument that a patient's right to know and to be informed should override any traditional professional distinctions on who should be responsible for disclosure, concluded that there was a possible conflict between a strong view of patients' rights and the need of hospitals to maintain orderly channels of communication.

Kurtzman, Block, and Steiner-Freud study.   In the study by Kurtzman et al. (1985), mean attitude scores were high for all student groups, suggesting strong agreement with theoretical rights for patients. Fourth-year nursing students, as compared with first-year nursing students, showed a higher proportion of strong agreement for nine out of ten items. In regard to informed consent, a smaller proportion of nursing students, as compared to medical students, perceived the existing blanket consent procedure as adequate for protection of patients' rights. Fourth-year nursing students suggested the need for specific informed consent much more frequently than did the other groups. Fourth-year nursing students assigned responsibility for protecting patients' rights to nurses, doctors, hospital administration, and the patient/family with higher frequency than other student groups.

Results of t tests comparing differences between scores of student groups were confusing as presented in the text and table of the study. However, it appeared that the only statistically significant differences were between mean scores of first-year and fourth-year nursing students (df = 71, $t = 2.224$).

The investigators concluded that findings did not support rejection of null hypotheses related to differences in attitudes between first-year nursing and medical students and first-year and fourth-year medical students. The hypothesis that fourth-year nursing students would have more positive attitudes than first-year nursing students was supported. We agree with the investigators' warning to interpret findings cautiously, in that attitude scores among all groups were unexpectedly high, perhaps reflecting the lack of validity of the instrument. They also appropriately cautioned against assuming that differences between first-year and fourth-year nursing students were due to the fostering of patient advocacy attitudes by nursing education.

Summary and Discussion

The small convenience samples from narrowly defined populations limit the generalizability of these studies, but suggest the following:

1. As nursing students progress in educational programs, attitudes indicate strong advocacy for increased role responsibilities of nursing in information disclosure, adequate informed consent for patients, and a more interdisciplinary focus in protection of patients' rights.

2. The lack of valid and reliable tools to measure variables related to professional autonomy and ethical decision making are a serious limitation in increasing our understanding of these variables.

3. Further research is needed to clarify differences in attitudes of autonomy and advocacy, patients' rights,

and rejection of the traditional nursing role limitations for students in different types of educational programs and at different levels of the program.

Nursing student attitudes toward disclosure of information to patients, the rights of patients, nursing autonomy, and traditional role boundaries need to be further explored. As future research builds on these exploratory studies, employing a variety of methodologies with reliable and valid measurement tools, we will have a clearer understanding of these problems within the context of ethics in nursing education.

With this review and critique of Part III on "Research on Attitudes of Nursing Students and Faculty toward Ethical Issues" concluded, we now proceed to Part IV, which focuses on "Research on Ethical Values of Nursing Students and Faculty."

Part IV

Research on Ethical Values of Nursing Students and Faculty

In this section of the monograph, we include studies related to ethical values of nursing students and faculty. The nine studies reviewed represent a wide range of topics, including studies which compared nursing students' values over time; nursing students' values with those of faculty; values of nursing students in secular schools with those in nonsecular schools; and values of nursing students with those of students in other disciplines. The values described in some of the studies would not ordinarily fall under the rubric of ethical values. Therefore, through mutual agreement, we focus here on the values typically categorized as ethical, for example, caring, equality, human dignity, and justice. Due to the differing focuses and cross-focuses evident in the studies reviewed here, we chose not to arrange the studies in subgroups, but to review them as a whole.

RESEARCH ON ETHICAL VALUES
IN EDUCATION

Of the nine studies we reviewed on values, three focused on values of undergraduate students and faculty (O'Neill, 1973, 1975; Thurston, Flood, Shupe, & Gerald, 1989). It is unclear whether the two studies by O'Neill (1973, 1975) were different aspects of the same study. The sample size differed for the two studies, but this could be due to inclusion of faculty in one study (1975). Garvin (1976) compared values of male and female nursing students and other groups. Studies by Schank and Weis (1989) and Blomquist, Cruise, and Cruise (1980) compared values of students in secular and nonsecular nursing programs. Garvin and Boyle (1985) compared values of two sets of students entering nursing, with a ten-year span between them. Williams, Bloch, and Blair (1978) focused on changes of students' values after one year of graduate study in nursing. Self (1987) studied the values of nurses and nursing students related to ethical decision making.

Conceptualization

Only one study (Self, 1987) specifically described the conceptualization of values within a framework of ethical theory. Self used a framework of value theory, noting that all ethical decisions are based on either complete subjectivism, partial subjectivism-partial objectivism, or complete objectivism. Self (1987) examined the various positions of nurses and nursing students in the subjective-objective controversy, determining whether value judgments are purely personal expressions of an individual's opinion, or whether these judgments emanate from an external value structure.

Although the other studies did not specifically describe values within a framework of ethical theory, there was some consistency in conceptualizations of values. Several investigators (e.g., Garvin, 1976; Garvin & Boyle, 1985; O'Neill, 1973, 1975; Williams et al., 1978) drew on conceptualizations of values from fields outside of nursing, citing studies in the literature of sociology, psychology, and education.

Two recent studies (Schank & Weis, 1989; Thurston et al., 1989) based their studies on values concepts derived from nursing documents. Schank and Weis (1989) measured values of subjects according to the ANA *Code for Nurses,* using the rationale that this Code was derived from the value system of the providers of nursing services, and that it identified the values that form the basis for professional standards of nursing practice and for ethical decision making. Thurston et al. (1989) defined values within the framework of the Rokeach Values Survey and the Seven Essential Values outlined in a 1986 report by the American Association of Colleges of Nursing (AACN). The AACN values were seen as essential values that baccalaureate nurses should possess upon graduation. Blomquist et al. (1980) cited the work of Rokeach as the central framework for their study.

We found that the lack of a common conceptualization of ethical values across these studies was a problem in critiquing the studies within a framework of ethics in nursing education. Investigators appeared to assume that the values measured were related to ethics, but except for Self (1987) did not use a theoretical framework of ethical theory. Garvin and Boyle (1985) defined values in broad terms, viewing them as general standards that guide behavior. They described these standards in relation to an individual's wants, needs, interests, beliefs, and attitudes. Williams et al. (1978) at times appeared to use the terms *values* and *attitudes* interchangeably. We believe that future studies of values in nursing education would be strengthened by a clearer conceptualization of the values being measured.

Purpose

Most of the studies reviewed had clearly stated purposes. Self (1987), noting the lack of studies of actual data gathered on the theoretical foundations of ethical decision making, stated an intent to identify the various philosophical positions of nurses and nursing students and the consistency of these positions with respect to ethical decision making. In one section, this intent was stated in terms of philosophical positions which these nurses and nursing students *utilize,* whereas the term *hold,* used in the abstract of the report, appeared to reflect more accurately the purpose of the study, since perceptions, not behaviors, were measured.

O'Neill (1973, 1975) identified a purpose of comparison of values of nursing students with those of other student groups. For the latter study, she also stated a purpose of comparison of values of nursing students with those of faculty.

Williams et al. (1978) stated four purposes: (a) determine the change occurring in graduate nursing students' values after one year of study, (b) determine variables influencing the extent of change in students' values, (c) describe graduate nursing students' values at admission and after one year of study in relation to values of graduate faculty, and (d) explore the influences of certain educational experiences and personal influences on change in values.

In the study by Thurston et al. (1989), the primary purpose was to explore values held by nursing faculty and to compare these findings with an earlier study of values held by nursing students at the same university. A secondary purpose was to determine faculty commitment to the seven values outlined in the AACN report.

Schank and Weis (1989) described their purpose as (a) an exploration of the impact of the type of educational experience, that is, secular or nonsecular nursing program, on the development of values, and (b) exploration of the values of the respondents of these educational programs in relation to values reflected in the ANA *Code for Nurses.*

Blomquist et al. (1980) stated a purpose of comparing values of students in secular and religious nursing programs. They also sought to determine if values of baccalaureate nursing students changed during their educational experiences.

The stated purpose of Garvin (1976) was to examine selected aspects of male nursing students' values. Garvin and Boyle (1985) stated their purpose as an examination of selected values of entering nursing students and a comparison of these findings with a similar study conducted ten years earlier (Garvin, 1976).

When viewing the purposes across studies, it is evident that all but Self (1987) identified a purpose of comparing values between groups. For Garvin and Boyle (1985), this comparison was between two groups of nursing students at different points in their educational program. The other investigators identified purposes of comparing nursing students with other types or levels of students, with faculty, with different types of educational programs, and/or with other health professionals.

Methods

Design. All of the studies used written questionnaires to obtain data. Self (1987) collected descriptive data on one group of nurses and nursing students without differentiating findings between the two groups. The other studies used designs in which values between groups were compared. Garvin and Boyle (1985) collected data on selected values of two groups of students at points in time that were ten years apart. Blomquist et al. (1980) were the only investigators who specified their research design as experimental, but it lacked characteristics of randomization and a control group.

Sample. All of the studies were based on convenience samples of students, faculty, and/or nursing graduates. Self (1987) submitted questionnaires to 912 nurses (RNs and LPNs) and 195 nursing students from one health care center, and received 381 responses, a return rate of only 34.4%. The nursing students, who comprised 46.5% of the sample, were at various stages in their educational programs. Since the presentation of data did not differentiate between nurses and nursing students, we found it difficult to interpret findings in relation to nursing education considerations.

O'Neill (1973) used the term *population* and *sample* interchangeably, stating that the 465 baccalaureate students from three nursing programs were the subjects who comprised the study population. O'Neill (1975) used a sample of 507 freshmen, sophomore, junior, and senior students and faculty from three baccalaureate nursing programs in the midwest. O'Neill noted that considerations of variation in size and whether private or state-supported were factors in selection of the institutions. However, no information was provided about the number of students versus faculty in this sample.

Williams et al. (1978) used a sample of 75 newly admitted graduate nursing students in one educational program who completed pretests and posttests at the end of one academic year. Twenty-two out of a possible 23 graduate faculty of the educational program served as the faculty sample. These faculty completed questionnaires only once, at the end of the academic year, based on an assumption by the investigators that the faculty members' values, perceptions, and expectations were relatively stable.

The study sample (n = 199) of Schank and Weis (1989) included 138 senior baccalaureate nursing students and 61 graduate nurses of a large secular and large nonsecular university. The senior students were surveyed approximately three months before graduation. The graduate nurses were surveyed from one to five years after graduation. It was not stated whether some of the graduate nurses were currently enrolled in graduate study in nursing. There was considerable discrepancy between educational levels in the two groups. In the secular group, 22% of graduate nurses had master's degrees; in the nonsecular group, only 1% had master's degrees. The majority of respondents in both groups were Catholic.

Thurston et al. (1989) included in their sample faculty and undergraduate nursing students from one university school of nursing. Fifty-four of a potential 79 faculty members volunteered as subjects. Student data were obtained from an earlier study by the investigators, which included 351 students who were enrolled in upper-division courses of a generic nursing program. Twenty percent of these students held baccalaureate or higher degrees in other disciplines, and ages ranged from 19 to 54.

The sample for the study by Blomquist et al. (1980) included 1,009 freshmen and senior baccalaureate nursing students. The investigators' description of the selection of this sample was confusing. They stated that the sample was drawn from students at three secular and four religious universities, but in describing the procedure for the study, they referred to only four universities. Registered nurses returning to school for a baccalaureate degree and nursing students with a baccalaureate degree in another field were specifically excluded from the sample. The majority of subjects were females between 20 and 30 years of age.

Garvin (1976) did not differentiate between study population and sample. Subjects included 34 male nursing students who entered a nursing program at different points in time, and 841 female nursing students from the same school.

Garvin and Boyle (1985) included in their sample one group of students entering a school of nursing in 1972 ($n = 309$) and one group entering the school in 1982 ($n = 161$). Demographic characteristics were not presented, but the investigators stated that comparison of demographic data did not reveal significant differences between the two groups for any demographic variable except education; significantly higher levels of education were reported for mothers of students in the second group.

Instruments.   The use of a variety of different instruments for the studies added to the complexity of evaluating the measurement of nursing/faculty values. In addition, due to the brief description of each of these values measured by an instrument, we found it difficult to ensure content validity related to defining traits of each instrument. However, in order to emphasize those study results most applicable to ethical values and to make some comparisons across studies, we attempted to identify for each study certain values that could be categorized as ethical values.

Self (1987) used a nine-item questionnaire which was developed specifically for the study. We determined that all nine questions were accurate reflections of ethical values, for example, the greatest good, right versus wrong, and ethical obligations. The questionnaire included three questions related to each of the three possible positions in the subjective-objective issue in value theory. Self stated that the questions were constructed in pairs in order to check for consistency in responses; this statement was confusing, in view of the inclusion of three questions for three separate positions, and the odd number of total questions. No information was provided on validity or reliability of the instrument, even though the instrument was adapted from one used in a similar study of physicians and medical students.

Garvin (1976), Garvin and Boyle (1985), and O'Neill (1973, 1975) used the Allport-Vernon-Lindzey Study of

Values (AVL) to measure values categorized as: theoretical, economic, aesthetic, social, political, and religious. The primary value for our emphasis was that of social, which was viewed in relation to love in its altruistic or philanthropic aspects. None of these investigators provided specific information about validity and reliability of the AVL, although Garvin and Boyle (1985) noted that value studies of nursing students have frequently used the AVL and that validity and reliability have been demonstrated.

Gordon's Survey of Interpersonal Values (SIV) was used by O'Neill (1973, 1975) and Williams et al. (1978). Gordon's Survey of Personal Values (SPV) was used by Williams et al. (1978). Williams et al. (1978) noted that the SIV and SPV instruments measure broad interests, not values, so that the use of the term *values* appeared to be a semantic convenience. The investigators provided information about standardization processes for the SIV and SPV and stated that reliability for all scales on the tests by both the test-retest method and the Kuder-Richardson formula were above 70; we assume the investigators meant .70.

The SIV measures the relative importance in a given personality of six values: support, conformity, recognition, independence, benevolence, and leadership. Of these values, we selected support, independence, and benevolence as being most clearly identified as ethical values. The SPV measures traits of: practical mindedness, achievement, variety, decisiveness, orderliness, and goal orientation. We determined that these traits were not closely associated with ethical values.

In addition to the SIV and SPV instruments, Williams et al. (1978) used two investigator-constructed questionnaires. These instruments were designed to obtain data related to demographics, influences of certain program and personal factors, goal orientation, and anticipated and actual outcomes. No information was presented about validity or reliability of the tool.

Blomquist et al. (1980) and Thurston et al. (1989) used Rokeach's Value Survey to assess instrumental and terminal values of respondents. Instrumental values are preferable modes of conduct; characteristics such as courageous, forgiving, helpful, honest, independent, loving, and responsible seemed most closely related to ethical values. Terminal values are desired end-states of existence; characteristics determined to be most reflective of ethical values were a world at peace, equality, freedom, mature love, and true friendship.

Blomquist et al. noted that only predictive validity had been reported by Rokeach for the instrument. Seven weeks after testing, test-retest reliability was found to be in the .70s. Thurston et al. (1989) cited a reference by Rokeach in which established content validity was discussed, and stated previous test-retest reliability as .87 for terminal values and .60 for instrumental values using a paired comparison method. The investigators also carried out reliability analysis for their modified version of the Rokeach instrument and, using Cronbach's alpha, obtained .84 for instrumental values and .79 for terminal values.

Thurston et al. (1989) also incorporated into their instrument the AACN Seven Essential Values. This instrument categorizes values as altruism, equality, aesthetics, freedom, human dignity, justice, and truth. All of these values except aesthetics were seen as appropriate for analysis as ethical values. Although the investigators noted that face validity of the AACN Seven Essential Values instrument was established by the AACN work group developing the instrument, we question the adequacy of only this type of validity for research studies. The investigators carried out reliability analysis for the revised format of the AACN tool and obtained an alpha coefficient of .94. They stated that no attempt was made to obtain retest data to establish internal consistency, but we assume that they meant stability of the instrument and not internal consistency.

Schank and Weis (1989) used a two-part questionnaire that they apparently designed. The first part asked respondents to identify their professional values with a single, open-ended question. The second part of the questionnaire was used to obtain sociodemographic data. Senior students were asked to answer 11 items, whereas the graduates were asked to respond to 25 items. Although data were analyzed in relation to how values of respondents were related to values reflected in the ANA *Code for Nurses,* the relationship of items in the instrument to values in the Code was not clearly stated.

Data Analysis, Results, and Conclusions

Self study. The presentation of results in this study (Self, 1987) made it difficult to relate findings to responses on the instrument. Only percentages of affirmative and negative responses to questions on the instrument were provided, and the relationship of each question to objectivism or subjectivism was not specified until the discussion section.

Hypotheses for the study were twofold: (a) nurses tend to be objectivist in value theory and (b) nurses are consistent in the philosophical foundations of their ethical decision-making. Self (1987) stated that analysis of the data required that both hypotheses be "rejected as not true" (p. 87), but did not state the type of statistical analysis used to reach this conclusion.

Another limitation in the study was the failure to differentiate between values of nurses and nursing students. We question Self's apparent assumption that responses of both of these groups would be similar. This assumption appears unwarranted in view of other studies of values discussed here. In discussing conclusions of the study, Self was careful to emphasize that the inconsistency of nurses' responses to questions about ethical questions found in this study should not be interpreted to mean that nurses are inconsistent in actual ethical decisions.

O'Neill studies. Analysis of variance with a .05 level of significance was used by O'Neill (1973, 1975) to measure differences between mean scores on values for groups. O'Neill (1975) stated that Spearman's rank-order correlation was also used in analysis of data. Due to lack of detail concerning the instrument, scoring of the instrument, and variables tested, however, the presentation of results in the report was sometimes unclear. Also, the lack of any tables in the report added to the difficulty of differentiating between various reported statistical analyses.

In both studies by O'Neill (1973, 1975) significant differences were found between nursing students' values when compared with values of students in other fields. Nursing students scored significantly higher on Social Value scores than students in other fields. However, O'Neill (1973, 1975) did not state that students other than nursing students were included in her sample. Her conclusions regarding comparison of nursing students with students in other fields were apparently based on value norms for students in other fields presented in the Allport-Vernon-Lindzey test manuals.

Significant differences in nursing students' values tended to decrease at successive class levels within each institution (1973, 1975), as did student/faculty value differences (1975). O'Neill (1973, 1975) discussed findings in relation to implications for nursing education, noting the need to plan meaningful learning experiences for students in order to reinforce desired values.

Williams, Bloch, and Blair study.   In this study, Williams et al. (1978) reported testing eight hypotheses with either the two-sample or paired t test, using $p = <.05$ as the level of significance. Selected results were as follows: (a) graduate students showed a significant increase in posttest scores on values of support and independence, and a significant decrease in posttest scores on the value of benevolence; and (b) there was no significant difference in extent of change in values between those students 26 years or younger and those 27 years or older.

The investigators noted that the increase in valuing of support and independence and the decrease in valuing of benevolence found with nursing students in this study were similar to changes in values of medical students seen in previous research. They suggested that socializing factors may operate within nursing and medical schools that differ from socializing factors in other disciplines, although little comparative data were available.

The investigators noted that a decrease in valuing of benevolence was not unexpected for undergraduate nursing students, who might be very idealistic about service to others upon entry into their program, but this assumption was not related to previous data. The investigators appeared more unsure about how to interpret the decrease in valuing of benevolence for graduate students. They offer a plausible explanation, noting that graduate students' pretest scores for this value were higher than pretest scores for faculty; thus these scores may have been inflated with the enthusiasm of beginning a new professional endeavor. The investigators concluded that, to a large extent, nursing students and faculty shared similar values.

Thurston, Flood, Shupe, and Gerald study.   For their study, Thurston et al. (1989) analyzed data with *t* tests, analysis of variance, and Duncan's multiple comparison test to answer four research questions. Results indicated that (a) frequencies for professional (AACN) values held by nursing faculty were greatest for human dignity and altruism; (b) frequencies for personal (Rokeach) values held by nursing faculty related to instrumental values were greatest for responsible, honest, and loving, and those related to terminal values were greatest for inner harmony, self-respect, and sense of accomplishment; (c) frequencies for personal (Rokeach) values held by students related to instrumental values were greatest for loving, honest, and responsible, and those related to terminal values were greatest for sense of accomplishment, happiness, and self-respect; and (d) faculty were significantly more committed to the AACN values than to the Rokeach instrumental and terminal values ($p = <.01$).

In discussing findings of the study, the investigators appeared to go beyond the data in suggesting that findings of the high value placed on human dignity by nursing faculty refuted the lack of respect by which nurses are often portrayed in the media. An alternative explanation that was not given was that preferred values are not always operationalized in practice. Although characteristics of justice, truth, and altruism were not ranked among the top three choices by faculty, the investigators noted that this may be explained by problems in sensitivity of the instrument in relation to each characteristic. Although not mentioned by the investigators, we found it interesting that frequencies of the top three choices by both faculty and students on Rokeach terminal values did not reflect those values most clearly related to ethics, for example, equality or freedom.

As in the study by Williams et al. (1978), Thurston et al. (1989) concluded that overall, values of nursing students and faculty were similar. Thurston et al. suggested further research on the impact of nursing curriculums on values and the effects of socialization of students into the nursing role. We agree with their recommendation that pencil-and-paper commitment to values needs to be compared with overt behaviors.

Blomquist, Cruise, and Cruise study. For the study of Blomquist et al. (1980), means were computed on the 36 Rokeach values by class level and school orientation. Two-way analysis of variance was done on each value to determine the influence of class level or school orientation. Differences were found between students in religious and secular schools for 25 values, with significant F-values ranging from 3.91 to 153.26. Differences were also found between freshmen and senior nursing students for 17 values, with significant F-values ranging from 5.42 to 27.60. The interaction effect of school orientation and class level of students was significant for only seven values; F-values ranged from 4.27 to 11.74.

Senior students, regardless of school orientation, ranked both the instrumental values of independence and honesty and the terminal value of freedom significantly higher than freshmen students ($p < .005$). Students from secular schools rated values of independence and freedom significantly higher than students from religious schools ($p < .005$). Students from religious schools valued honesty significantly more than students from secular schools ($p < .05$). The investigators noted that a surprising finding was that freshmen valued helpfulness significantly higher than senior students ($p < .005$).

We found the investigators' discussion of results helpful in their relation of findings to values seen as ethical values. They also stated suggestions for further research in nursing education, including the use of a longitudinal design to measure changes of students' values over time and the use of other instruments to measure values.

Schank and Weis study. In this study, Schank and Weis (1989) and a research assistant independently analyzed open-ended responses on the first part of the questionnaire with content analysis. Interrater agreement exceeded the preestablished criterion of 90%. Analysis was not described clearly in relation to interpretive statements of the ANA *Code for Nurses.* Frequency distributions and means were used to compare respondent groups. Although the investigators stated that multivariate procedures were used to test for significance where differences were noted, the types of procedures, alpha levels, and calculated statistics were not presented, making it difficult to interpret validity of conclusions.

The investigators presented findings according to the six research questions. Professional values of respondents were coded into 12 categories, which included ethical values such as caring, helping, respect for the individual, patience, honesty, loyalty, and accountability/responsibility. No significant differences in value identification were found between respondents from secular and nonsecular nursing programs. The value most frequently identified by students (80%) correlated with the first statement in the ANA *Code for Nurses* that related to respect for human dignity and the uniqueness of the client; the value most frequently identified by graduates (92%) correlated with the fourth statement in the ANA *Code for Nurses* that related to responsibility and accountability. Eighty-five percent of the graduates also identified values related to the first statement in the ANA Code. No significant differences were found in value statements between students and graduates from either secular or nonsecular programs.

In view of the limitations imposed by the instrument design, as noted by the investigators, as well as the limited sample from only two universities, we question the investigators' conclusion that graduates of educational programs have not fully developed the value orientation of the profession, especially as related to social issues, embodied in the ANA *Code for Nurses*. We agree with their suggestion that further research is needed to identify if social values can be internalized by students before graduation, or whether these must come from involvement in professional practice.

Garvin study. In this study, Garvin (1976) did not state clearly the rationale for use of both one-way analysis of variance and the student's t test to test differences between mean scores of groups, and only results with t values were presented. Male nursing students scored significantly higher than female nursing students on the theoretical scale and significantly lower on the religious scale. The significance levels provided for these two scales were inconsistent, with a level of $p < .01$ for the theoretical scale stated in the text and a level of $p < .001$ stated in the table. For the religious scale, the text stated a significance level of $p < .001$, whereas the table stated this level as $p < .01$. Male nursing students scored significantly higher ($p < .001$) than general male collegiate norms on economic and political scales and significantly lower ($p < .01$) on the aesthetic and social scales. Garvin discussed her findings in relation to implications for nursing education, noting the high value scores of male students and the need to increase the awareness of high school counselors of the potential which men have for positive contributions to nursing.

Garvin and Boyle study.   Chi-square analysis was used by Garvin and Boyle (1985) to compare demographic variables of two groups of entering nursing students with a ten-year span between them. No significant differences between the two groups (1972 and 1982 groups) were found for age, sex, marital status, hometown size, or father's education. Mothers of students in the 1982 group had significantly higher levels of education than those in the 1972 group. The alpha level was not provided for this data, but the .01 alpha level was used for other data analysis.

The student's t test was used to compare mean scores on each of the six scales of the AVL instrument for both the 1972 and 1982 groups. No significant differences were found on the theoretical, aesthetic, social, political, or religious scales. The 1982 group scored significantly higher on the economic scale.

Spearman's rho was used to compare the rank order of the scales. For both groups, the social scale ranked highest, and the aesthetic and religious scales ranked in the top three for both groups. A Spearman rank-correlation coefficient of .77 was obtained. Garvin and Boyle (1985) discussed various implications of their findings, noting aspects that did or did not support findings of previous studies, and considered possibilities for the lack of change in value orientations. In recommending further research, the investigators noted the sexist nature of several of the AVL test items, and recommended that the AVL be revised to eliminate this problem.

Summary and Discussion

A review of these studies suggests the following:

1. Current state of studies of the concept of values as related to nursing education is still in an exploratory

stage. Differing conceptualizations of values among researchers and the lack of a common conceptualization of ethical values creates difficulty in comparing studies within a framework of research on ethical values.

2. Instruments used to measure values of nursing students/faculty are also in the exploratory stage of development. Most of the instruments used did not differentiate specific values as ethical values.

3. Present studies do not consistently differentiate values of nursing students and faculty.

4. Present studies suggest that nursing students undergo changes in values in the educational process, but the specific variables leading to these changes and the relationship to ethical decision making are poorly defined.

5. Most research of values of nursing students up to this time has concentrated on undergraduate students. Only one study was located that measured value changes in graduate nursing students.

6. Up to the present, investigators have used written questionnaires to measure values. In order to relate values to ethical decision making, future research is needed to evaluate values through observation of nurses in actual classroom and clinical situations.

As the complexity of the health care environment and the nurse's role increase dramatically, the ethical values of the nurse are critical in decision making related to patient care. Although there is much discussion related to this concern, little empirical research has been carried out to identify whether values of nursing students/faculty are congruent with professional codes and standards, or to identify factors in the educational process that strongly influence development of ethical values in students.

We have completed our discussion and critique of the individual empirical studies related to research on ethics in nursing education. We now move on to address conclusions, implications, and recommendations drawn from all of the studies discussed in Parts II, III, and IV of the monograph.

Part V

Summary

In this section, we formulate conclusions based on the 39 studies we reviewed in the monograph. From these conclusions, we then draw implications and recommendations for nursing education practice and nursing education research.

CONCLUSIONS, IMPLICATIONS, AND RECOMMENDATIONS

In the body of this monograph, we categorized similar types of studies into Parts II, III, and IV and then described, integrated, critiqued and discussed them. In Part V, we determine commonalities of content and method across the 39 studies and then formulate conclusions. The conclusions serve as the bases for implications and recommendations for nursing education practice and nursing education research.

Conclusions

We found drawing conclusions from the 39 studies difficult due to the following factors: (a) overall, the independent and/or dependent variables focused on a wide variety of areas; (b) the sample sizes and types varied; (c) in some areas, few studies were available for review; and (d) methodological problems and mathematical errors raised doubts about the validity of some results. Nevertheless, despite these limitations, we offer the following tentative conclusions, which we have divided into two categories: (a) content conclusions that focus on the subject matter and (b) methodological conclusions that focus on the research process.

133

Content conclusions.   Regarding content, the following major conclusions were drawn from the reviewed studies:

1. Overall, since the mid-1970s, steady progress has occurred in incorporating ethics content into nursing curriculums.

2. The results of studies that focused on the effects of ethics instruction on students' level of moral development or behavior were inconclusive. However, there appears to be a beginning trend that ethics courses or ethics instructional strategies increased some aspects of students' ethical awareness.

3. Both nursing students and nursing faculty engaged in unethical classroom and clinical behaviors.

4. A consistent and positive relationship occurred between students' unethical classroom and unethical clinical behaviors.

5. During the 1970s, when the attitude toward abortion studies included in this review were conducted, Catholic nursing students consistently held less favorable attitudes toward abortion than did other students.

6. Studies on nursing students' attitudes toward AIDS, toward aggressiveness of nursing care for terminally ill patients, and toward patient rights, as well as nursing studies on ethical values, were so diverse that no conclusions could be drawn with one tenuous exception: both nursing students and nursing faculty highly valued respect for human dignity.

7. Investigators have not conducted research that focuses on values as an ethical concept.

Methodological conclusions.   Regarding research methods, the following major conclusions were drawn based on the reviewed studies:

1. Overall, the vast majority of reviewed studies tended to be atheoretical. Even when a theoretical or conceptual framework was used, it was rarely integrated throughout the study.

2. Study purposes tended to be significant and clearly stated.

3. The vast majority of study designs were descriptive.

4. In the vast majority of reviewed studies, sampling techniques were inadequately described, randomization was rare, and rationales were only given occasionally for sampling decisions.

5. Regarding instrumentation, the following trends occurred: (a) investigators usually used appropriate instruments to measure their study variables; (b) investigators were inconsistent in describing their instruments and how they were scored; (c) investigators were inconsistent in reporting validity and reliability data; and (d) investigators tended to use surveys, questionnaires, and case studies.

6. Overall, data analysis techniques were appropriately selected, although rarely were rationales given for the selection, and levels of measurement were often ignored. In some studies, presentation of results was confusing because the results either did not answer the research questions, or the results included data for which there were no research purposes.

7. The following problems regarding conclusions surfaced in several studies: (a) conclusions were not stated; (b) conclusions did not relate appropriately to the research purposes; or (c) conclusions went beyond the presented results.

In addition to the above conclusions, we offer additional observations. First, virtually all the studies were short-term, with few studies building on one another. If more than one article by an author existed, it tended to be a derivative article including data from a larger study, or a derivative article using the same data but for a different audience. Second, the majority of articles were published in nonresearch journals. Third, the majority of articles published in research journals occurred during the 1970s and were articles on either attitudes or values. Fourth, few interdisciplinary studies were conducted. Fifth, scientific writing was often unclear, making critiquing of the articles difficult. However, despite these limitations, the overall picture regarding this review is one that reflects investigators' ability to discern significant research topics on ethics in nursing education, to accept diversity regarding ethical studies in nursing education, and to increase research efforts in this area.

Implications

Implications are discussed both for nursing education practice and nursing education research.

Nursing education practice.   Although progress has been made in incorporating ethics into nursing curriculums, more can be done. Several of the investigators of the reviewed studies concluded that gaps do remain both in ethical content and in ethical decision making in nursing education. From our own experiences, we have observed that these gaps too often cause not only an inadequate knowledge base for students and faculty but also a loss of their self-confidence in dealing with ethical issues.

We found a tentative, yet encouraging, trend from the reviewed studies that changes in the curriculum and/or instructional strategies can increase students' level of moral development or ethical decision making. This trend suggests that faculty can be active participants in bringing about curricular or classroom teaching strategies that facilitate students' growth in the area of ethics. Fortunately, faculty today have a wide variety of ethics books, audiovisual materials, and experts to assist them with this goal.

That some nursing students and nursing faculty engage in unethical classroom and clinical behaviors is disconcerting. Although realistically we can expect a small percentage of unethical behavior in any profession, nurse educators must try to understand the underlying basis for the behavior. For example, our own experiences have shown that both students and faculty are often unclear about some aspects of unethical behavior, for example, what constitutes plagiarism. Communication at both faculty and student levels is essential to arrive at clear definitions and examples of ethical and unethical behaviors *before* problems occur. We commend those investigators who have studied this problem; however, further research is needed to increase nursing faculties' and students' awareness of the nature and complexity of the problem.

Virtually every author of a current textbook on ethics stresses that values influence one's ethical position and, thus, one's ethical decisions. Yet, we found little empirical research on this concept; and this research tended to focus on specific traits, for example, honesty. This approach seems premature; we must first understand the meaning of the term *values* and its implication for ethical decision making before significant research questions on the topic can be raised. This understanding is critical because an ethical dilemma often involves a conflict of values, and the resolution of the dilemma may not occur until the value conflict is resolved. Thus, students should be introduced to scholarly works that define and conceptualize the nature of values and how to resolve value conflicts before attempting to conduct much needed values research related to ethics in nursing education.

Nursing education research. The overall quality of research we reviewed on ethics in nursing education could have been improved by: (a) increased ability to conceptualize and integrate frameworks throughout the research studies, (b) increased opportunities for obtaining knowledge about the research process, (c) enhanced opportunities to practice scientific writing, (d) increased attention to details that comprise scholarliness, and (e) increased opportunities for constructive peer review. Each of these factors, which we discuss in the following section, has implications for students, educators, investigators, and consumers of nursing research.

We respect the right of nurse educators to use different approaches in teaching research. We also recognize that controversies over content and teaching methods exist; however, certain basics are essential for a study to have scientific merit. For example, we become concerned when the majority of research on any significant body of knowledge in nursing is atheoretical, as was the situation here. This is not to say that *every* research study should be grounded in theory, but, overall, the advancement of nursing science is impaired if theory appropriate to the study purposes does not guide research. In addition, none of the reviewed studies displayed the integration of theory throughout, and none of the studies were theory-generating or theory-testing studies.

Another concern of ours was the investigators' lack of justification of their methodological decisions. Investigators described their studies, but rationales related to sample size or sampling techniques, research design, data analysis, and so forth, typically were not given.

Effective scientific writing is a learned skill that is grounded in knowledge and takes practice. Many of the studies we reviewed lacked clarity, conciseness, and readability. As a result, in our critiquing role, we sometimes felt frustrated. Were the methodological problems that we noted a result of inadequate knowledge, unclear thinking, practical constraints, compromises, typographical errors, or an inability to communicate clearly in writing? Of the six preceding conjectures, the latter one is usually the easiest to correct, but opportunities must exist to correct the problem through scientific writing experiences in nursing curriculums or through continuing education courses.

In addition to the problem with scientific writing, we were also concerned about the number of mathematical and other scholarship errors we detected in these studies. Too often, numbers did not add up, wrong numbers from probability tables were used, inconsistencies in dates were reported in different sections of an article, titles in the bodies of the articles were inaccurate, information in the references was incorrectly cited, and dates in the text and in the references were not consistent. As nurse educators, we need to stress the importance of accuracy, of checking every detail, of relying on more than one source to ensure accuracy, and of our personal and professional accountability to produce a quality research product.

One mechanism to help overcome the preceding problems is peer review. These reviews occur between faculty and faculty, faculty and students, students and students, and investigators and outside peer reviewers. This process of constructive critique results in a higher quality and, thus, a more scholarly product. Each person involved in the conduct and writing of research must internalize the concept of objectivity, that is, the development of the ability to remove oneself from one's own work and assess it from the prospective consumer's point of view. Professional maturity is attained when investigators can accept the results of a constructive critique with genuine appreciation. We believe that the concept of peer review and its ultimate rewards should be stressed in nursing curriculums, particularly in the difficult area of scientific writing for research.

Recommendations

Recommendations are identified both for nursing education practice and nursing education research.

Nursing education practice. Regarding nursing education practice, the following recommendations based on the reviewed studies are suggested:

1. Schools of nursing should systematically assess their curriculums for ethics content, including research on ethics. This content should be appropriate to the course material, reflect increased depth when indicated, and include topics essential for both graduate and undergraduate students.

2. Schools of nursing should ensure that students have clinical experience in actual, and not only hypothetical, ethical decision-making situations.

3. Faculty should identify teaching strategies based on research that best prepare students to cope with ethical issues in their professional practices.

4. Faculty should implement policies and procedures to deal with unethical colleague and student behaviors *before* they occur.

5. Faculty should assist students to define and conceptualize the nature and meaning of ethical values so that this concept can assist students with the resolution of ethical conflicts.

Nursing education research. Regarding nursing education research, the following recommendations based on the reviewed studies are suggested:

1. Nationally recognized representatives from educational and other appropriate groups should convene to develop a comprehensive and systematic short- and long-term plan for research on ethics in nursing education. A variety of research related to ethics in nursing education such as historical research, concept analysis research, theory-generating research, and theory-testing research should be considered. In addition, priorities for ethics in nursing education research should be established.

2. Schools of nursing should critically examine the adequacy of their curricular content at all levels related

to research, as well as their own preparedness to meet the highest standards of excellence regarding the conduct of research.

3. Schools of nursing should include in their curriculums information on scientific writing that begins at the baccalaureate level and continues through the doctoral level. Furthermore, students should have many and varied opportunities to practice this style of writing.

4. Schools of nursing should also concern themselves with the socialization of students and faculty into the research role. Student and faculty investigators must understand that the final scientific and ethical accountability for the quality of their research rests with them.

5. *Current* studies related to nursing students' attitudes toward abortion should be encouraged; other studies needed for replication purposes so that conclusions can be drawn include nursing students' attitudes toward AIDS, patients' rights, and aggressiveness of nursing care for terminally ill patients.

6. Investigators should consider interdisciplinary approaches to research on ethics in nursing education.

7. Investigators should more widely disseminate their research on ethics in nursing education to include *both* research and nonresearch journals that have an interest in educational ethics.

In summary, during the 1970s and early 1980s, investigators began conducting research on ethical issues in nursing education. By the mid-1980s to the present, research in this area has increased substantially. We hope that this integrated review and critique of the preceding 39 studies will serve as a useful guide for assessing the progress we have made, the problems we have to solve, and the challenges we have yet to discover in this important area of nursing.

We cannot close Part V without mentioning an important resource for persons interested in research on ethics. That resource is dissertation abstracts. To that end, Part VI presents dissertation abstract key concepts by author and titles on research on ethics in nursing education.

Part VI

Dissertation Abstract Key Concepts, Authors, and Titles on Research on Ethics in Nursing Education: A Bibliography

Rose M. Chop, MN, RN, and
Carolyn K. Lewis, MSN, RN

In Part VI, we include a bibliography of dissertation abstract key concepts, authors, and titles on research on ethics in nursing education. To accomplish this goal, we conducted extensive searches using several data bases and hand searches. We then formulated a systematic protocol to select the dissertation abstracts that specifically focused on the topic of research on ethics in nursing education.

INTRODUCTION

The purpose of this section is to provide the reader with a comprehensive collection of dissertation abstract titles specific to research on ethics in nursing education both by authors and by key concepts. To locate dissertation abstracts on ethics in education, two data bases were searched: Dissertation Abstracts International and On-Line Computer Library Center. As noted in Part I, 1970 through 1990 was the search period for the computer data bases, including the dissertation abstracts. In addition, hand searches were conducted on relevant bibliographies and integrative reviews from 1985 through 1990 to obtain current dissertation abstracts that the Dissertation Abstracts International search did not locate. Even though the data bases were searched through December of 1990, some abstracts that were published in the latter part of the year may not be indexed until later into 1991 and thus do not show up in this bibliography. Although there may be other significant unpublished research investigating ethics in nursing education, we used only dissertation abstracts because of (a) the availability of a centralized data base from which to concentrate our search and (b) the large amount of research related to ethics in nursing education in Dissertation Abstracts International.

147

To assess validity and reliability for the selection of dissertation abstract titles, as well as the categorization of key concepts, the following protocols were used:

1. Interrater reliability for "Dissertation Abstract Key Concepts by Author" was established by one of the primary monograph authors and the authors of Part VI. There was 88% agreement on author placement for the concepts. Validity for "Dissertation Abstract Key Concepts by Author" was obtained by one of the primary monograph authors; she read the dissertation abstracts for key concepts to determine the accuracy of author placement for the concepts. One of the limitations noted was the difficulty of developing mutually exclusive categories for key concepts of dissertation abstracts. Validity for "Dissertation Abstract Titles by Author" was obtained by the same primary monograph author to ensure that the selected dissertation abstract titles accurately reflected the topic of "research on ethics in nursing education." Some of the abstract titles may seem misleading because they do not reflect the nursing education component in the title; however, in reviewing the abstract, the key words noted in Part I were included in the dissertation abstracts selected.

2. Reliability for "Dissertation Abstract Titles by Author" was obtained by the authors of Part VI who (a) reviewed the bibliographies and integrative reviews separately and then cross-referenced each others' dissertation abstracts from the reviews for 100% interrater reliability; (b) reviewed the computer data bases separately and then cross-referenced the searches for relevance to the monograph purpose for 95% interrater reliability; and (c) provided a rationale, if a disagreement occurred, to either accept or reject the dissertation abstract.

The remainder of Part VI is subdivided in two sections. The first section is entitled, "Dissertation Abstract Key Concepts by Author." Each author is listed alphabetically under the respective key concept; however, because of the content of the abstract, an author may appear under more than one key concept. The second section is entitled, "Dissertation Abstract Titles by Author." The content, which typically reflected itself in the dissertation abstract titles, specifically focused on research on ethics in nursing education. In addition, each author is noted and each reference is cited according to the year it was published in Dissertation Abstracts International.

DISSERTATION ABSTRACT KEY CONCEPTS

By Author

AUTONOMY
Aronovitz, F. B.
Benner, M. P.

COGNITIVE/MORAL DEVELOPMENT
Aronovitz, F. B.
Awtrey, J. S.
Beardslee, N. Q.
Bell, S. K.
Bridston, E. O.
Crisham, P.
Edgil, A. E.
Felton, G. M.
Fleeger, R. L.
Frisch, N. C.

COGNITIVE/MORAL DEVELOPMENT (cont.)
Giovinco, G.
Hembree, B. S.
Henderson, M. C.
Holzman, P. G.
Jamison, M.
Johnson, R. W. H.
Kellmer, D. M.
Kennedy, P. H.
Munhall, P. L.
Roell, S. M.
St. Denis, H. A.
Slomowitz, A. M.
Thomas, P. A.
Valiga, T. M. G.

ETHICAL INSTRUCTIONAL
  STRATEGIES
Bell, S. K.
Biehler, B. A.
Bridston, E. O.
Frisch, N. C.
Gilbert, C.
Hembree, B. S.
Henderson, M. C.
Hilliard, M. T.
Kellmer, D. M.
Kennedy, P. H.
Krawczyk, R. M.
Obester, D. M.
Payton, R. J.
St. Denis, H. A.
Turner, S. L.
Walters, M. L.

ETHICAL VALUES
Agrafiotis, P. C.
Benner, M. P.
Blair, E. L.
Bornhauser, H. M.
Cerato, K. J.
Frisch, N. C.
Kelly, B. O.
Shehata, S. Z. A.
Uustal, D. B. T.
Walters, M. L.

MORAL COMPETENCE
Benner, M. P.

MORAL/ETHICAL DILEMMA
Crisham, P.
Dison, N. J.
Eberhardy, J. L.
Felton, G. M.
Hembree, B. S.
Winland-Brown, J. E.

MORAL JUDGMENT
Aronovitz, F. B.
Crisham, P.
Edgil, A. E.
Krawczyk, R. M.
Winland-Brown, J. E.

MORAL/ETHICAL REASONING
Awtrey, J. S.
Beardslee, N. Q.
Bridston, E. O.
Felton, G. M.
Fleeger, R. L.
Hembree, B. S.
Henderson, M. C.
Holzman, P. G.
Jamison, M.
Kennedy, P. H.
Munhall, P. L.
Mustapha, S. L. W.
Roell, S. M.
St. Denis, H. A.
Swanson, J. V.
Turner, S. L.
Winland-Brown, J. E.

DISSERTATION ABSTRACT TITLES

By Author

Agrafiotis, P. C. (1988). An analysis of the curriculum of moral education of baccalaureate nursing students in New England. *Dissertation Abstracts International, 49,* 360B. (University Microfilms No. 88-07,502)

Aronovitz, F. B. (1985). Autonomy, socialization, strength of religious belief and socioeconomic status as predictors of moral judgement in associate degree nursing students. *Dissertation Abstracts International, 46,* 112B. (University Microfilms No. 85-06,550)

Awtrey, J. S. (1981). Moral reasoning of baccalaureate nursing students. *Dissertation Abstracts International, 41,* 4453B–4454B. (University Microfilms No. 81-12,733)

Beardslee, N. Q. (1984). Survey of teaching ethics in nursing programs and the investigation of the relationship between extent of ethics content and moral reasoning levels. *Dissertation Abstracts International, 44,* 2380B–2381B. (University Microfilms No. 83-24,326)

Bell, S. K. (1985). Effect of a biomedical ethics course on senior nursing students' level of moral development. *Dissertation Abstracts International, 45,* 3205B–3206B. (University Microfilms No. 84-29,854)

Benner, M. P. (1985). Value pluralism, moral competence, and nursing education. *Dissertation Abstracts International, 46,* 643A. (University Microfilms No. 85-11,222)

Biehler, B. A. (1987). Using instructional design to resolve a problem in teaching ethics to baccalaureate nursing students. *Dissertation Abstracts International, 47,* 3959A. (University Microfilms No. 87-05,737)

Blair, E. L. (1973). A study of students' values in three university programs in nursing. *Dissertation Abstracts International, 33,* 3740B–3741B. (University Microfilms No. 73-17,54)

Bornhauser, H. M. (1978). A study of baccalaureate nursing student values in a church-related college. *Dissertation Abstracts International, 38,* 3902A. (University Microfilms No. 77-29,308)

Bridston, E. O. (1979). The development of principled moral reasoning in baccalaureate nursing students. *Dissertation Abstracts International, 40,* 1237A. (University Microfilms No. 79-20,589)

Cerato, K. J. (1985). The effects of a graduate nursing curriculum on the professional value systems of students. *Dissertation Abstracts International, 45,* 3528A. (University Microfilms No. 85-02,630)

Crisham, P. (1980). Moral judgment of nurses in hypothetical and nursing dilemmas. *Dissertation Abstracts International, 40,* 4212B. (University Microfilms No. 80-06,598)

Dison, N. J. (1986). Dilemmas of baccalaureate nursing students. *Dissertation Abstracts International, 46,* 3390B. (University Microfilms No. 85-26,469)

Douglas, J. L. (1986). Ethical content in baccalaureate nursing curricula. *Dissertation Abstracts International, 46,* 2621B. (University Microfilms No. 85-22,551)

Eberhardy, J. L. (1983). An analysis of moral decision making with nursing students facing professional problems. *Dissertation Abstracts International, 43,* 3542A. (University Microfilms No. 83-08,040)

Edgil, A. E. (1981). Variables related to the principled level of moral judgment of nurses. *Dissertation Abstracts International, 41,* 4455B–4456B. (University Microfilms No. 81-12,734)

Felton, G. M. (1985). Attribution of responsibility, ethical/moral reasoning and the ability of undergraduate and graduate nursing students to resolve ethical/moral dilemmas. *Dissertation Abstracts International, 46,* 474B–475B. (University Microfilms No. 85-08,176)

Fleeger, R. L. (1986). Critical thinking and moral reasoning behavior of baccalaureate nursing students. *Dissertation Abstracts International, 47,* 1915B–1916B. (University Microfilms No. 86-16,530)

Frisch, N. C. (1987). The value analysis model and the moral and cognitive development of baccalaureate nursing students. *Dissertation Abstracts International, 47,* 2467A. (University Microfilms No. 86-22,978)

Gallo, A. M. (1985). Nursing curriculum theorizing and its application to practice: A critical analysis. *Dissertation Abstracts International, 46,* 1511B. (University Microfilms No. 85-15,378)

Gilbert, C. (1980). Ethics and its application to nursing: An experimental study with baccalaureate nursing students utilizing an engineering design with a specific learning program. *Dissertation Abstracts International, 40,* 5374A. (University Microfilms No. 80-07,871)

Giovinco, G. (1986). Using patient care situations to apply Kohlberg's moral development theory to nursing. *Dissertation Abstracts International, 46,* 2333A. (University Microfilms No. 85-21,084)

Hembree, B. S. (1989). The effect of moral dilemma discussions on moral reasoning levels of baccalaureate nursing students. *Dissertation Abstracts International, 50,* 494B. (University Microfilms No. 89-09,782)

Henderson, M. C. (1988). Effect of empathy training on moral reasoning and empathic responding of nursing students. *Dissertation Abstracts International, 49,* 352B. (University Microfilms No. 88-04,997)

Hilliard, M. T. (1987). The identification of nursing ethics content and teaching strategies for baccalaureate nursing curriculum through policy delphi. *Dissertation Abstracts International, 48,* 52A–53A. (University Microfilms No. 87-10,266)

Holzman, P. G. (1985). A comparative study of liberal arts and nursing students' moral development in collegiate programs. *Dissertation Abstracts International, 45,* 3772B. (University Microfilms No. 85-02,589)

Jamison, M. (1981). Lawrence Kohlberg's theory of moral development: The impact of peer pressure on moral reasoning and behavior. *Dissertation Abstracts International, 42,* 1177B. (University Microfilms No. 81-19,162)

Johnson, R. W. H. (1980). A comparison of the perceptions among student nurses from associate degree, baccalaureate and diploma programs in nursing about the influence of significant others and the curriculum upon the moral/ethical component of the professional role. *Dissertation Abstracts International, 41,* 521B. (University Microfilms No. 80-18,423)

Kellmer, D. M. (1984). The teaching of ethical decision making in schools of nursing: Variables and strategies. *Dissertation Abstracts International, 45,* 1732B. (University Microfilms No. 84-16,265)

Kelly, B. O. (1988). Perception of professional ethics among senior baccalaureate nursing students. *Dissertation Abstracts International, 49,* 693B. (University Microfilms No. 88-04,060)

Kennedy, P. H. (1990). Curricular approaches to ethical instruction and the development of moral reasoning in baccalaureate nursing students. *Dissertation Abstracts International, 50,* 2370A–2371A. (University Microfilms No. 89-17,028)

Krawczyk, R. M. (1982). Moral judgement level of nursing students in three different nursing programs. *Dissertation Abstracts International, 43,* 380A. (University Microfilms No. 82-15,657)

Krizinofski, M. T. L. (1985). A conceptual foundation for nursing ethics. *Dissertation Abstracts International, 45,* 3468B. (University Microfilms No. 85-01,715)

Mahon, K. A. (1981). Constructs used by registered nurses in ethical decision making: The development of an instrument. *Dissertation Abstracts International, 42,* 1600A–1601A. (University Microfilms No. 81-20,481)

Munhall, P. L. (1980). Moral reasoning levels of nursing students and faculty in a baccalaureate nursing program. *Dissertation Abstracts International, 40,* 4216B–4217B. (University Microfilms No. 80-06,842)

Mustapha, S. L. W. (1986). An examination of moral reasoning in college students in two types of general education curricula: Implications for nursing education. *Dissertation Abstracts International, 47,* 428A. (University Microfilms No. 86-08,467)

Obester, D. M. (1986). The place of ethics as an area of study in the curricula of schools of nursing in Pennsylvania. *Dissertation Abstracts International, 47,* 1624A. (University Microfilms No. 86-17,243)

Payton, R. J. (1979). A bioethical program of study for baccalaureate nursing students. *Dissertation Abstracts International, 39,* 6625A–6626A. (University Microfilms No. 79-10,311)

Penny, J. T. (1983). A comparison of faculty and nurse practitioner opinions regarding practice issues, political education, and professional ethics. *Dissertation Abstracts International, 44,* 404A. (University Microfilms No. 83-14,196)

Preheim, G. G. (1985). Perspectives in psycho-ethical decision making: Implications for collaboration between nursing education and practice. *Dissertation Abstracts International, 46,* 1872B. (University Microfilms No. 85-14,220)

Roell, S. M. (1982). Moral development levels of university educated graduate and undergraduate nursing students. *Dissertation Abstracts International, 43,* 736A–737A. (University Microfilms No. 82-17,286)

St. Denis, H. A. (1980). Effects of moral education strategies on nursing students' moral reasoning and level of self-actualizing. *Dissertation Abstracts International, 40,* 6078A–6079A. (University Microfilms No. 80-11,047)

Schilling, M. J. (1979). Ethics in the curriculum of schools of nursing in Texas: A function of selected administrative and institutional characteristics. *Dissertation Abstracts International, 40,* 1122B–1123B. (University Microfilms No. 79-20,381)

Shehata, S. Z. A. (1981). Perceptions of student nurses and registered nurses of the value of general education. *Dissertation Abstracts International, 41,* 4300A. (University Microfilms No. 81-06,896)

Slomowitz, A. M. (1982). The relationships of graduate training in psychotherapy, moral development, and ego development. *Dissertation Abstracts International, 42,* 4591B. (University Microfilms No. 82-01,054)

Swanson, J. V. (1990). Ethical reasoning among baccalaureate female nursing students. *Dissertation Abstracts International, 50,* 2754A–2755A. (University Microfilms No. 90-05,364)

Thomas, P. A. (1990). Cognitive development in a traditional and nontraditional nursing student population. *Dissertation Abstracts International, 51,* 2822B–2823B. (University Microfilms No. 90-32,094)

Turner, S. L. (1991). An evaluation of the effectiveness of a guided design instructional package on ethical decision-making of senior nursing students. *Dissertation Abstracts International, 51,* 3762B–3763B. (University Microfilms No. 91-00,737)

Uustal, D. B. T. (1983). Values education in baccalaureate nursing curricula in the United States. *Dissertation Abstracts International, 43,* 3857A. (University Microfilms No. 83-10,342)

Valiga, T. M. G. (1982). The cognitive development and perceptions about nursing as a profession of baccalaureate nursing students. *Dissertation Abstracts International, 43,* 1447A. (University Microfilms No. 82-23,179)

Walters, M. L. (1980). An experimental study of the impact of a program on the medical options of sanctity of quality of life upon nursing students. *Dissertation Abstracts International, 41,* 954A. (University Microfilms No. 80-20,454)

Winland-Brown, J. E. (1984). A comparison of student nurses, nurses and non-nurses with regard to their moral judgments on nursing dilemmas. *Dissertation Abstracts International, 44,* 3362B. (University Microfilms No. 84-03,838)

Zablow, R. J. (1985). Preparing students for the moral dimension of professional nursing practice: A protocol for nurse educators. *Dissertation Abstracts International, 45,* 2501B. (University Microfilms No. 84-24,277)

REFERENCES

Armiger, B. (1977). Ethics of nursing research: Profile, principles, perspective. *Nursing Research, 26,* 330–336.

Aroskar, M. A. (1977). Ethics in the nursing curriculum. *Nursing Outlook, 25,* 260–264.

Aroskar, M., & Veatch, R. M. (1977). Ethics teaching in nursing schools. *The Hastings Center Report, 7*(4), 23–26.

Blomquist, B. L., Cruise, P. D., & Cruise, R. J. (1980). Values of baccalaureate nursing students in secular and religious schools. *Nursing Research, 29,* 379–383.

Carmack, B. J. (1984). Exploring nursing educators' experience with student plagiarism. *Nurse Educator, 9,* 29–33.

Cassells, J. M., Redman, B. K., & Jackson, S. S. (1986). Generic baccalaureate nursing student satisfaction regarding professional and personal development prior to graduation and one year post graduation. *Journal of Professional Nursing, 2,* 114–127.

Cassells, J. M., & Redman, B. K. (1989). Preparing students to be moral agents in clinical nursing practice: Report of a national study. *The Nursing Clinics of North America, 24,* 463–473.

Cassidy, V. R., & Oddi, L. F. (1988). Professional autonomy and ethical decision making among graduate and undergraduate nursing majors. *Journal of Nursing Education, 27,* 405–410.

Chally, P. S. (1990). Moral and ethical development research in nursing education. In G. M. Clayton & P. A. Baj (Eds.), *Review of*

Research in Nursing Education (Vol. 3, pp. 33–47). New York: National League for Nursing.

Davis, A. J., & Jameton, A. (1987). Nursing and medical student attitudes towards nursing disclosure of information to patients: A pilot study. *Journal of Advanced Nursing, 12,* 691–698.

Elder, R. G. (1975). Attitudes of senior nursing students toward the 1973 Supreme Court decision on abortion. *Journal of Obstetric, Gynecology, and Neonatal Nursing, 4*(4), 46–54.

Felton, G. M., & Parsons, M. A. (1987). The impact of nursing education on ethical/moral decision making. *Journal of Nursing Education, 26,* 7–11.

Fischer, E. H. (1979). Student nurses view an abortion client: Attitude and context effects. *Journal of Population, 2*(1), 33–46.

Frisch, N. C. (1987). Value analysis: A method for teaching nursing ethics and promoting the moral development of students. *Journal of Nursing Education, 26,* 328–332.

Garvin, B. J. (1976). Values of male nursing students. *Nursing Research, 25,* 352–357.

Garvin, B. J., & Boyle, K. K. (1985). Values of entering nursing students: Changes over 10 years. *Research in Nursing & Health, 8,* 235–241.

Gaul, A. L. (1987). The effect of a course in nursing ethics on the relationship between ethical choice and ethical action in baccalaureate nursing students. *Journal of Nursing Education, 26,* 113–117.

Gaul, A. L. (1989). Ethics content in baccalaureate degree curricula: Clarifying the issues. *The Nursing Clinics of North America, 24,* 475–483.

Gortner, S. R. (1985). Ethical inquiry. *Annual Review of Nursing Research, 3,* 193–214.

Hilbert, G. A. (1985). Involvement of nursing students in unethical classroom and clinical behaviors. *Journal of Professional Nursing, 1,* 230–234.

Hilbert, G. A. (1987). Academic fraud: Prevalence, practices, and reasons. *Journal of Professional Nursing, 3,* 39–45.

Hilbert, G. A. (1988). Moral development and unethical behavior among nursing students. *Journal of Professional Nursing, 4,* 163–167.

Hurwitz, A., & Eadie, R. F. (1977). Psychologic impact on nursing students of participation in abortion. *Nursing Research, 26,* 112–120.

Ketefian, S. (in collaboration with I. Ormond). (1988). *Moral reasoning and ethical practice in nursing: An integrative review.* New York: National League for Nursing.

Ketefian, S. (1989). Moral reasoning and ethical practice. *Annual Review of Nursing Research, 7,* 173–195.

Killeen, M. L. (1986). Nursing fundamentals texts: Where's the ethics? *Journal of Nursing Education, 25,* 334–340.

Kurtzman, C., Block, D. E., & Steiner-Freud, Y. (1985). Nursing and medical students' attitudes toward the rights of hospitalized patients. *Journal of Nursing Education, 24,* 237–241.

Lawrence, S. A., & Lawrence, R. M. (1989). Knowledge and attitudes about acquired immunodeficiency syndrome in nursing and non-nursing groups. *Journal of Professional Nursing, 5,* 92–101.

Lewandowski, W., Daly, B., McClish, D. K., Juknialis, B. W., & Youngner, S. J. (1985). Treatment and care of "do not resuscitate" patients in a medical intensive care unit. *Heart & Lung, 14,* 175–181.

Munhall, P. (1980). Moral reasoning levels of nursing students and faculty in a baccalaureate nursing program. *Image, 12,* 57–61.

Mustapha, S. L., & Seybert, J. A. (1989). Moral reasoning in college students: Implications for nursing education. *Journal of Nursing Education, 28,* 107–111.

O'Neill, M. F. (1973). A study of baccalaureate nursing student values. *Nursing Research, 22,* 437–443.

O'Neill, M. F. (1975). A study of nursing student values. *International Journal of Nursing Studies, 12,* 175–181.

Pinch, W. J. (1985). Ethical dilemmas in nursing: The role of the nurse and perceptions of autonomy. *Journal of Nursing Education, 24,* 372–376.

Rosen, R. A. H., Werley, H. H., Ager, J. W., & Shea, F. P. (1974a). Health professionals' attitudes toward abortion. *Public Opinion Quarterly, 38,* 159–173.

Rosen, R. A. H., Werley, H. H., Ager, J. W., & Shea, F. P. (1974b). Some organizational correlates of nursing students' attitudes toward abortion. *Nursing Research, 23,* 253–259.

Schank, M. J., & Weis, D. (1989). A study of values of baccalaureate nursing students and graduate nurses from a secular and a nonsecular program. *Journal of Professional Nursing, 5,* 17–22.

Self, D. J. (1987). A study of the foundations of ethical decision-making of nurses. *Theoretical Medicine, 8,* 85–95.

Shelley, S. I., Zahorchak, R. M., & Gambrill, C. D. S. (1987). Aggressiveness of nursing care for older patients and those with do-not-resuscitate orders. *Nursing Research, 36,* 157–162.

Swider, S. M., McElmurry, B. J., & Yarling, R. R. (1985). Ethical decision making in a bureaucratic context by senior nursing students. *Nursing Research, 34,* 108–112.

Theis, E. C. (1988). Nursing students' perspectives of unethical teaching behaviors. *Journal of Nursing Education, 27,* 102–106.

Thurston, H. I., Flood, M. A., Shupe, I. S., & Gerald, K. B. (1989). Values held by nursing faculty and students in a university setting. *Journal of Professional Nursing, 5,* 199–207.

Wertz, D. C., Sorenson, J. R., Liebling, L., Kessler, L., & Heeren, T. C. (1987). Knowledge and attitudes of AIDS health care providers before and after education programs. *Public Health Reports, 102*(3), 248–254.

Wiley, K., Heath, L., & Acklin, M. (1988). Care of AIDS patients: Student attitudes. *Nursing Outlook, 36,* 244–245.

Williams, M. A., Bloch, D. W., & Blair, E. M. (1978). Values and value changes of graduate nursing students: Their relationship to faculty values and to selected educational factors. *Nursing Research, 27,* 181–189.

Winder, A. E., & Stanitis, M. A. (1988). Nuclear education in public health and nursing. *American Journal of Public Health, 78,* 967–968.

Winget, C., Kapp, F. T., & Yeaworth, R. C. (1977). Attitudes towards euthanasia. *Journal of Medical Ethics, 3,* 18–25.